MINERALS

An authoritative gui
of the most importa
recognize deficiency
sufficiency of these

MINERALS
What They Are and Why We Need Them

by

MIRIAM POLUNIN

NATURE'S WAY

THORSONS PUBLISHERS LIMITED
Wellingborough, Northamptonshire

First published 1979
Second Impression 1980

ISBN 0 7225 0528 0 (hardback)
ISBN 0 7225 0524 8 (paperback)

Photoset by
Specialised Offset Services Ltd., Liverpool.
Reproduced, printed and bound in Great Britain
by Cox & Wyman Ltd., Reading.

CONTENTS

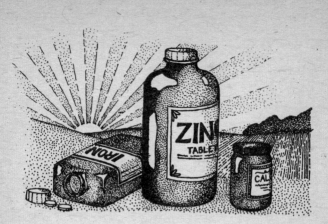

INTRODUCTION

What is a mineral? A dictionary definition is 'a solid homogenous crystalline chemical element or compound that results from the inorganic processes of nature'. For many people, minerals mean the iron, nickel, tin and other metals that are industry's raw materials. It is only in the last twenty years that the other role of minerals has been fully appreciated: as the vital raw materials for *us*.

Although iron, calcium, iodine and a few other minerals have been recognized as being necessary to human health for several decades, nobody paid much attention to all the other minerals in our environment. Vitamins were being discovered and given their deserved importance, but minerals played Cinderella in the background.

Now minerals are exciting the medical and biochemical worlds. It is as though a big door had opened, through which lie many useful discoveries about human health and healing. It is now clear that minerals are just as important as vitamins, in fact, almost more important; for while the body can manufacture some vitamins for itself, it is *completely dependent* on outside sources – food, drink and air – for all its minerals. And 'all' means far more minerals than used to be thought essential.

Over twenty different minerals are now recognized as being necessary to man – and a few more may yet be added to that number. Some are metals, others are not. *Without the right amounts of each, basic body functions are thwarted.* The exploration of how minerals work, how much of each we need, and what illnesses may be caused by lack or excess of them is now in full swing.

THREE MAIN FUNCTIONS

The three main groups of functions for which minerals are needed are:

1. As basic material for bones and teeth (e.g. calcium, phosphorus and magnesium).
2. As 'triggers' for enzyme processes in the body, processes which are vital to every cell. This is the main purpose of most minerals.
3. As controllers of the balance, amount and composition of body liquids, inside and outside our cells: the function of sodium and chlorine in the fluids outside the cells; of potassium, magnesium and phosphorus inside the cells.

DISREGARD OF MINERALS

Why have minerals been so neglected until now? There are several reasons. The first concerns attitudes. Many of the minerals we need are present in the body in very tiny amounts – thousandths of a gram in some cases. It seems to be human nature to concentrate on, and be impressed by, the larger things in life. For a long time, a common view was that such miniscule amounts of substances in the body could not be very important. This was in spite of the fact that our bodies contain a far larger total amount of minerals than they do of vitamins.

The average adult has about seven pounds of minerals in the body – elements we share with the plants, water, stones, earth and other animals of our world. When the Bible says 'the Lord God formed man out of the dust of the ground', it speaks with authority.

But the only minerals that man thought of studying carefully were the ones which are present in large amounts – such as sodium, phosphorus and calcium – and the ones whose deficiency symptoms happened to be discovered early – iron and iodine.

The second reason was that methods for detecting the presence of minerals, especially the ones present in such tiny amounts that they are known as 'trace' elements, were poor.

A third reason was chance. Much of our knowledge about nutrition has been acquired by historical accident. It was the painful experience of sailors on long voyages that led to interest being focused on the importance of what they ate, and then on vitamin C. In a similar way, it has mainly been examples of mineral-deficient communities and areas which have pushed forward our investigations into the functions of minerals. Chronic mineral deficiencies in the soil of an area will affect the food and health of the whole community living there – making the condition obvious. It is a perfect research opportunity which cannot be produced deliberately.

NEW INTEREST IN MINERALS

Now the interest in all minerals is intense. And the spotlight on the tiny, trace elements is as bright as on the better known minerals – because size is no longer seen as the factor determining importance. Small may be vital for minerals, just as we have accepted it is with vitamin B12, despite the fact that it is needed in such small amounts that the daily requirement for the whole of Britain fits into a small medicine bottle.

The present investigations would not be possible had not methods of identifying and measuring minerals been enormously improved. But the treasure chest of mineral knowledge has only been opened a crack so far. So is there anything of use to the non-scientist, the ordinary person interested in improving or maintaining their own personal well-being?

Yes, there is. Curiously enough, it is ordinary people who are jumping in and using the new knowledge about minerals as fast as it is published – often well before it is put to practical use by the medical profession.

A VITAL ROLE

Minerals are not magic medicines, but they are vital parts of our diet. There are many circumstances where they may be missing from the food we eat, or lost to us before our bodies can use them. If they are not available to our bodies in the right balance, form and amount, our health suffers. Supplying such deficiencies by taking mineral supplements is a growing practice among health-conscious people – and one which is likely to increase within a few years.

But as with most things in life, you can have too much of a good thing. Many essential minerals are good for health in small amounts but thoroughly dangerous in very large quantities. A few minerals are 'baddies' through and through: they serve no useful purpose for man, and only have ill-effects when we are exposed to them.

This book aims to put you ahead of the game, so that you can be sure that minerals are playing the role they should in your life.

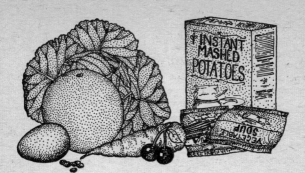

CHAPTER ONE

ARE WE GETTING ENOUGH?

Minerals are parts of food and drink, just like vitamins, fats, proteins, carbohydrates or fibre. And just as with all these other nutrients, the conventional attitude is 'Don't worry. If you eat a well-balanced diet, you'll get plenty of everything.'

But what is a well-balanced diet? And how do you judge if yours *is* well balanced? We live in an age where, for the first time, everyone has enough money to exercise a good deal of choice about what they eat. For the first time, therefore, people choose what they feel like eating, rather than choosing only what they can afford to eat. And, at the same time, because of modern transport and storage methods, they have a new, immense variety of foods from which to choose.

THE CONSEQUENCES OF FREEDOM
We all know from daily observation what an extraordinary range of eating habits has resulted from this freedom: the supermarket trolley next to yours which is laden with foods you never eat, the weight-watcher who feels happiest with endless

grapefruits and cottage cheese salads, the teenager who seems to live on chocolate bars.

We certainly have plenty to eat, in terms of quantity. Most of us, according to figures showing that about half of us should lose some weight, have too much. This is not the same as saying that we are eating a well-balanced diet – or getting enough minerals. It is quite possible to be over-fed, in calorie terms, but seriously under-nourished.

There are several ways in which this can happen with minerals.

CHOOSING BADLY

Many people choose an unbalanced range of foods. It is often thought that people have an instinctive urge towards the foods their body needs. Perhaps very young children do. But most of us choose the food we eat for reasons that have very little to do with instinct: for instance, habit, regional origin, belief that a certain food has certain properties, social conditioning, nostalgia and advertising.

Habit begins early, with our parents as they choose our food for us. If they are used to eating cabbage, we soon are too. If they believe that 'greens give me indigestion', greens are likely to be a novelty to us. If we are Scottish, we will be used to eating far more bread and cakes; or, if we were brought up in the North, to drinking more tea in relation to coffee.

Social conditioning is an even more powerful shaper of eating habits as we grow up. Children have little sense of what is 'correct' to eat at what meal – fish fingers for breakfast are quite acceptable to them. But by the time we are fifteen, we are thoroughly indoctrinated with the conventions of what constitutes breakfast food – and revealing that you eat potato crisps for breakfast is likely to make your friends think you distinctly odd.

OUTSIDE INFLUENCES

Every year, as we grow up, our tastes are shaped by outside influences: a school which murders cauliflower by over-cooking it to a pulp may put a generation of pupils off cauliflower for life. An imagination-catching advertising campaign for a breakfast cereal may give it a lifelong standing in the affections of the children who saw those advertisements.

People's basic eating habits are firmly formed by the age of twenty, and changes after then are likely to be through circumstances (such as moving to another country, or needing to lose weight) rather than through choice. And those tastes, as I have suggested, are closely linked with emotional roots – region, family, childhood memories.

No, instinct does not get much of a look in. And the food most people seem to choose certainly does not appear to be what their bodies would be asking for anyway.

CALORIES

If you think of our daily food as a budget of calories, we are 'spending' more and more of them on sweet, rich and processed foods.

In the last two hundred years, sugar and fat have become the cheapest and most popular sources of calories around. They are also the most calorie-laden foods we have. At 112 calories per ounce for sugar, and twice that amount per ounce for fat, they contain an amazingly high amount of calories in a small weight of food. An ounce of sugar, for instance, has almost the same number of calories as four ounces of cottage cheese; an ounce of butter, which we might easily tuck away in a single breakfast, has more calories than five apples.

In terms of mineral supplies, the trend has been unfortunate. For sugar – refined white sugar, which provides in food and drink about 20 per cent of all our energy – has no minerals to speak of at all. And fat – which provides over 40 per cent of our calories – provides only a very limited amount and range of minerals.

SUGAR AND FAT

'I hate fatty food and I hardly ever eat sweet things!'

If you find yourself saying this, just ask yourself whether, from time to time, you do not eat pastry, biscuits, *pâtés*, sausages, chocolate, cake, ice cream, potato crisps, or pies? All these foods are high – deceptively high – in fat. The reason we do not think we eat a lot of fat is because most of this kind of food is bought ready made. We do not see the basic ingredients – so we never realize how big a part fat plays – for instance in chocolate (about 40 per cent fat) or in pastry (about 33 per cent fat).

As for sugar, divide the amount available in Britain each year by the population, and you will find we each eat between four and five ounces a day. Again, it is not all visible spoonsful transferred from a packet or bowl: it is the sugar in cereal, in jam, in sweet drinks, in fruit dishes, in yogurts, or in milk puddings. Of course, there are other ingredients in these foods. Some of them are useful mineral sources – such as cereals, fruit, yogurt or meat. But the fact remains that by eating so many of our calories in sugar and fat, we eat fewer of other foods which contribute more valuable minerals.

National Food Survey figures show conclusively that no matter what we think we eat, nor how we picture the gluttonous dinners of the Victorian era, somehow or other, we eat more sugar and more fatty foods than people (excepting an affluent few) used to eat.

LOST IN TRANSIT

Besides the shift in the proportions of different foods which we eat, there has been another trend which has reduced our total mineral supply. This has been the inexorable development of food refining. For the last 150 years, the food industry has been perfecting methods of transporting food over long distances, between countries, and from farm to housewife, keeping it apparently in good condition throughout. But it has not perfected one aspect of this convenient skill. For to obtain long-lasting food that travels well, refining has been increased. And refining causes mineral (as well as other nutrient) reduction.

The main losses are from our staple foods, cereals. In the refining of wheat to make white flour, 30 per cent of the grain is removed. The white-versus-wholemeal bread argument often ignores the very large advantage of wholemeal bread and flour in mineral terms. In the removal of bran and wheat germ from flour, the following essential minerals are lost*:

Element	Wholewheat	White	Average % loss
Chromium, ppm	1.75	0.23	87
Cobalt, ppm	0.07 – 0.2	0.05 – 0.07	70
Copper, ppm	1.8 – 6.2	0.62 – 0.63	70 – 90
Iron, ppm	18 – 31	3.5 – 9.1	81
Magnesium, ppm	0.09 – 0.12	0.013 – 0.021	83
Manganese, ppm	24 – 37	2.1 – 3.5	91
Molybdenum, ppm	0.3 – 0.66	0.16 – 0.39	50
Selenium**	0.04 – 0.71	0.01 – 0.63	12 – 75
Zinc, ppm	21 – 63	3.9 – 10.5	83

ppm = parts per million, or ten thousandths of a per cent.

The flour in bread, pastry, biscuits, cakes, buns and other foods should be one of the most important sources of chromium, iron, magnesium, manganese and zinc. Iron is the only one of these added back to flour by law – and in recent years, it has been recognized that it is added back in a form in which the body probably cannot use it.

Calcium is also added to all flour except wholemeal and self-raising varieties by law. This is not so much because wholemeal flour is a rich calcium source (although it does contribute some of

* Figures for average wheat samples from H. Shroeder's *The Trace Elements And Man*, Deven-Adair, Old Greenwich, Conn., U.S.A.
** The selenium content of wheat varies enormously depending on the soil where the crop grew.

our calcium requirements) but for historical reasons. During the Second World War, when food needs were for the first time seriously planned and considered, it was feared that shortages of dairy foods, combined with the use of bread which had a higher than usual fibre content, might leave some people short of calcium. The phytic acid in wholemeal flour was thought to be a threat to calcium supplies, because it could combine with calcium in food and make it unavailable to the body. After the war, the practice was continued, even though it is now realized that most of the phytic acid in flour is broken down during dough fermentation in breadmaking; people who eat high phytic acid diets are not seen to have lower calcium levels than other people. But apart from its added calcium, white flour is clearly a mineral-deficient food.

The refining of rice and maize causes similar, substantial mineral losses. These are increasingly important since breakfast cereals – of which these grains are the basic ingredients – have become the main breakfast food of over 40 per cent of us over the last twenty years. Children are particularly dependent on breakfast cereals for their nutrient supplies. And in the past twenty years, white polished rice has become far more widely eaten with the combined influence of Chinese, Indian and other overseas cooking traditions.

FREEZING

Other refining processes also cause mineral losses: freezing, for instance. In many ways, freezing is the best method of food preservation we have. But the blanching that precedes the freezing of vegetables and fruit is liable to remove substantial amounts of their valuable calcium, manganese and zinc.

When frozen meat thaws, the liquid that drips from it may contain significant amounts of iron and other essential minerals. And the freezing of fish is now suspected of causing loss of iodine, the vital mineral of which sea food is one of the very few, and therefore important, sources.

SUGAR

Raw brown sugar contains substantial amounts of trace elements, which are almost completely removed in the subsequent processing to obtain white sugar. Molasses is far, far richer in minerals than any other 'sweet' product, with black treacle in between. But raw sugar only carries these beneficial elements with it if it is genuine West Indies raw sugar (the darker, the more mineral-rich), not 'London Demerara' which is white sugar with colouring.

Element	Raw	White	Blackstrap molasses	Black treacle
Calcium (mg)*	52	5	580	500
Chloride (mg)	35	trace only	1,200	80
Chromium (ug)**	30	9	27	27
Cobalt (ug)	40	under 5	125	
Copper (mg)	0.3	0.05	1.4	0.4
Iron (mg)	1-4	0.1	11.3	9
Magnesium (mg)	10-14	0.3	?	144
Phosphorus (mg)	19-44	1.0	85	31
Potassium (mg)	90-230	0.5	1500	1470
Sodium (mg)	6-24	0.3	80	10
Sulphur (mg)	14	trace only	?	68
Zinc (ug)	870	20	830	?

Minerals in sugar – average amounts per 100g (approximately 3½ oz.). Figures from Shroeder and others.

LOST FROM THE START

Processing nowadays often starts before harvest. The continual pressure to keep food prices as low as possible has encouraged farmers to adopt many new techniques to produce more food from less land and outlay. One such development has been the continuing trend from mixed farms to specialist farms, where the same land is used year after year for the same crop.

The soil contains elements which the crop feeds

* milligrams: 1g = 1000mg
** micrograms: 1mg = 1000ug

on. If different crops are grown, they require different elements. But if the same crop is grown repeatedly, the soil's supply of that crop's needs is exhausted. And farmers can no longer afford to leave a field lying fallow to recover its strength. Instead, the crop is fed with man-made and man-chosen fertilizers, which contain the nutrients known to be necessary for the crop to grow and yield as desired.

But, just as with humans, the trace elements which are needed in smaller amounts may be ignored. Unlike vitamins, minerals cannot be constructed by the plant itself. If they are not provided by soil or fertilizers, they will not be there in the finished product – the grain, seed, vegetable or fruit.

The extent to which the mineral content of harvested foods has changed has hardly been investigated so far, but where it has, the conclusions are not reassuring. Basic mineral sources for man – such as carrots – may not supply the minerals we expect from them, because they cannot collect them from mineral-bankrupt soil.

THE KITCHEN SINK

We can't blame all mineral losses upon other people. Many minerals go down the average sink or into the dustbin.

Most of them come from vegetables. We start by throwing away the outer leaves – the very part that is richest in minerals. We go on to peel off the mineral-rich outer layers of root vegetables. We soak away more minerals by leaving prepared vegetables in water. Finally, we reject the water in which the vegetables are cooked – and into which a significant proportion of their mineral value has leached.

To keep the maximum minerals, we should follow the same rules as for vitamins: use as much of the vegetable as possible; don't soak it, particularly if chopping has opened up a big surface area to the water; cook in the minimum of liquid for the minimum of time; and use the cooking liquid whenever possible as stock for sauces, soups or casseroles.

OUT OF BALANCE

The removal of a trace element or any other nutrient – oil, vitamin or enzyme – in food processing may have more effect than a simple loss of that element. This is because so many of our essential food elements are interdependent. Without one, another may not be able to function properly.

This is particularly likely in the case of minerals, since their main role is as part of enzymes, the protein substances that are needed as 'starters' for many of the body's processes. Losing chromium, for instance, may prevent the body dealing efficiently with the sugar we eat. Recently, this piece of knowledge has led to the successful use of chromium in the treatment of some cases of diabetes. In sufferers from diabetes, which is a disease of faulty sugar digestion, chromium levels are well below normal. By taking chromium, some test patients were able to reduce or dispense with insulin.

In natural, unprocessed, foods, the minerals and vitamins the body needs to digest and use that food efficiently are usually present together – as chromium is in sugar cane.

The result of processing may thus be deeper than appears. By losing the natural balance of the food, its whole value to our health may be jeopardized.

INDIVIDUAL NEEDS

We all recognize that some people seem to need far more food than others of the same age and build. The same applies to minerals. Some people are able to adapt more flexibly to changes in food supplies and do not seem to experience any change in health. Others are more vulnerable, perhaps because of genetic disposition, or because their general nutritional status is more precariously balanced to start with.

That is why whenever a group of people are in adverse nutritional circumstances – be it the siege of Leningrad or racing round the world in a small yacht – some will show ill-effects sooner than others.

The fact that your best friend drinks to excess, smokes and never bothers with sensible eating, yet feels fine, is no guarantee that you can do the same.

Vulnerabilities tend to run in families, for three reasons. The first is genetic. There are hereditary characteristics of metabolism as well as visible physique. The second is upbringing. Our daily living habits are often carried on from those of our family and if they omit a health-helping habit, such as eating fresh vegetables, the whole family may continue living in a vulnerable way. The third reason is geographical. Certain areas have nutritional characteristics of both culture and nature. The Scots, for example, normally eat far more flour-based foods than southern English people; people who come from Derbyshire are liable to iodine-deficiencies, because the soil in that area is naturally low in that element.

DEFICIENCY SYMPTOMS

For all these reasons, mineral deficiencies can occur in our apparently well-nourished society. Moreover, the tiny amounts of minerals we need do not mean that the effects of lacking them are slight. A daily shortage in childhood of a few millionths of an ounce of zinc, for instance, can lead to stunted growth or lack of normal sexual development. The total amount of zinc lost over the years could be contained in a lunchbox.

Other deficiency symptoms are far less easy to recognize – but they can still make life less easy to deal with. Mild anaemia, for example, is probably the vaguest and yet most common mineral deficiency so far recognized. Statements such as 'I don't seem to have any energy', 'I wake up as tired as when I went to bed' or 'I don't know why everything gets me down nowadays' are easy to write off as moodiness, or to blame on different circumstances. They could be due to a vitamin deficiency. But they could so easily, especially if the speaker is female, be iron-deficiency anaemia.

Who knows what other 'not ill, but not well' feelings could be simply solved by restoring minerals to food – instead of being dismissed as 'Neurotic – take some Valium'.

GETTING THROUGH

'But if we only need tiny amounts of minerals, surely a varied diet would supply them from something', you might feel. Which leads to the biggest problem in mineral supply – and one which is only now being fully appreciated.

To be available to the body, minerals not only have to enter our mouths in foods or supplements: they have to be absorbed into the blood from the digestive passage. The efficiency of this stage of digestion varies with the mineral, with the person and with the form in which the mineral is taken. And it is often so poor that even when large amounts of a mineral are taken, the body goes short.

Minerals that are by nature poorly absorbed include iron, calcium, copper, chromium, cobalt and manganese. In some cases, only a twentieth or less of the amount in food may be usable. Again, our individuality plays a part: some people are more efficient absorbers than others.

But much of our efficiency of absorption depends on the form in which the mineral is presented to the body. We have already mentioned the recent, reluctant, admittance that the iron added back to white flour and bread is in a form the body can barely use. That still leaves thirty years in which white bread has been smugly counted as a useful source of iron. The same happy illusion lay behind the rise – and fall – of Popeye, with his invigorating tins of spinach. In most people's eyes, 'spinach' is still almost as good as saying iron. But the form of iron in spinach is one the body cannot easily break down for the all-important transfer across the intestinal wall (though it is still a useful source of other food elements).

UNANSWERED QUESTIONS

The gradual growth of knowledge of the nature and behaviour of minerals has improved our judgement of which foods are best sources of which minerals, but there are still many questions unanswered. For instance, it is not understood why people who live in low calcium-intake countries (such as Japan) seem to be just as well off in calcium status as heavy calcium dairy produce eaters such as New Zealanders.

And while theoretical knowledge increases, practice may lag well behind. The average doctor uses only two minerals: iron and calcium. The first is given in vast amounts, much in a poorly absorbable form which produces uncomfortable digestive upsets and constipation. Calcium is given to thousands of old people in an attempt to halt the decalcification of bones many undergo. Yet it is already well established that calcium by itself will not do this job. Decalcification (which leads to brittle bones which fracture easily) depends on some interaction of nutrients which is not yet understood.

The future of minerals looks brighter and exciting. These tiny but powerful Cinderellas are about to become as respected as they deserve. Meanwhile, the information in this book can help you check that *you* are not neglecting this vital part of your health.

The following chapters discuss the uses and needs of all the minerals now thought to be essential to man. The harmful effects of the few dangerous minerals and of mineral overdoses are dealt with in the chapter *Mineral Overdoses* (page 85).

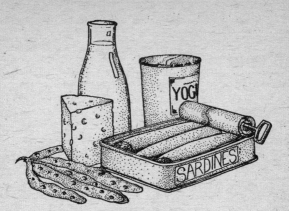

CHAPTER TWO

CALCIUM

Calcium is the mineral present in the largest quantity in the body – about 1200g, or over $2\frac{1}{2}$ lb in the average adult. Ninety-nine per cent of it is in our bones, where calcium compounds form the solid basis of our skeletons, and teeth.

Contrary to what one might imagine, bone is not a static, unchanging part of the body. There is a constant alteration even throughout adult life, although it does not show up as obviously as it does in a growing child. It is thought that about 700g of calcium enter and leave the bones every day. Even in an adult, therefore, the skeleton undergoes a complete renewal about once a decade. In a child, it is almost yearly.

Calcium is thus an essential raw material for this basic rebuilding, although it needs other elements – particularly phosphorus (see page 83) – and a favourable nutritional climate in the body to work properly.

The 1 per cent of calcium that is in our blood, not

our bones, has different important functions. It is essential for muscle contraction, and for blood clotting, and calcium determines the strength of nerve reactions to stimuli.

Besides these functions in which it is the main component, calcium also helps activate enzymes which are necessary to trigger off other body processes. For instance, calcium helps the body use iron; is necessary for the body's use of vitamin D; is necessary for parathyroid hormone to function. As with many food elements, much of our knowledge of the need for calcium is based on evidence of what happens without it.

INTAKE
The recommended daily intake in the United Kingdom is 500mg per day for adults, while babies up to the age of one are thought to need at least 600mg, and teenagers 700mg.

Americans are recommended to take 800mg per day for children and adults, up to 500mg for babies up to the age of one. During pregnancy or breast-feeding, this figure is increased to 1200mg in both countries. Breast-fed children need less calcium because they absorb more from this form.

Recommended calcium intake is designed to balance the natural daily loss of calcium from the body. This is via the urine and faeces, and, to a much lesser extent, through sweat. The daily output of calcium from the body is a mixture of calcium present in food eaten, but not absorbed; discarded cells which contain calcium, and used digestive juices. It varies considerably with the individual, but is usually within the range of 550 to 1000mg per day.

DEFICIENCY CIRCUMSTANCES
An inadequate supply of calcium for its essential body functions can occur for several reasons:

1. *Insufficient eaten*, due to eating patterns poor in calcium-supplying foods. Rich sources are

relatively few, although there are many foods which supply some calcium to the diet. Water's calcium content varies widely from area to area: it can be an important or a negligible source of the mineral. Hard water areas have a higher calcium content, with limestone or chalk soil areas contributing up to 200mg per day to the person who drinks water from the area. Soft water areas, such as peaty soil districts, may contribute too little to have any value. The average contribution in the United Kingdom is thought to be about 75mg per day.

Since the foods richest in calcium are dairy products, fresh green leafy vegetables and oily fish where the bones are eaten (such as sardines or whitebait), it is people who eat little of these who are most at risk: non-dairy eating vegetarians, people eating meals without green vegetable portions and those who for any reason are eating small amounts of food.

2. *Increased need* is most likely to occur in pregnant or breast-feeding women who pass on large amounts of calcium to the growing child. A pregnant or breast-feeding woman may pass on about 300mg of calcium a day to the baby, and this will be the same whether she is taking extra calcium or not. The mother is always the loser, not the child.

Lack of exercise increases the body's output of calcium – so those who are confined to bed for more than a day or two need extra. About 200mg per day more than usual may be lost.

Emotional turmoil is thought to increase the body's turnover of calcium.

People who are recovering from illness, operations or infections clearly need to have extra supplies of many nutrients for the speediest recovery – and this includes calcium. At these times, absorption of nutrients may be impaired, and calcium is particularly vulnerable to malabsorption.

3. *Poor absorption is almost normal* with calcium, with about three quarters of all calcium eaten in food failing to be absorbed. Absorption takes place

only in the presence of adequate oxygen and of some form of energy-giving fuel, such as glucose.

The poor absorption of calcium is not entirely understood, but some of the factors are known.

INFLUENCES ON CALCIUM ABSORPTION

Vitamin D is essential to calcium absorption by providing a 'carrier' substance at the intestinal absorption stage. An adequate intake of protein is also necessary to good calcium absorption, so that more is absorbed from high-protein foods such as dairy produce. However, a very high intake of protein – over 90g per day – may worsen calcium absorption.

Saturated fats, however, are also high in many protein foods, and the fatty acids in these may combine with calcium to form compounds which the body cannot break down to extract the calcium.

Oxalic acid, which is present in some fruit and vegetables, can restrict calcium absorption in the same way. Oxalic acid is high in tea, cocoa, rhubarb, spinach, beetroot, parsley and chocolate (from the cocoa). However, most people do not eat so much of these foods that they would make a serious dent in their calcium intake.

For many years, it was thought that two other substances could endanger the body's calcium supply: too high a level of phosphorus or phosphate compounds; and phytic acid, a phosphorus compound present in cereals, particularly in their outer layers. Like oxalic acid, the phytic acid can combine with calcium in food, forming calcium phosphate which, in theory, the body cannot absorb calcium from.

PHYTIC ACID

The phytic acid controversy began in 1925, when Mellanby showed that the calcium in wholemeal bread and oatmeal (both higher in phytic acid than white bread) was less absorbable by puppies than calcium in white bread. It happened that more tests confirming this effect were completed at the time in the Second World War when the 'National Loaf', which included more of the outer layers of the wheat, was being introduced. In view of the general restricted food situation, it was decided that extra calcium should be added to the National Loaf to offset any loss of calcium caused by the extra phytic acid.

This has been practised ever since: by law, 14 oz. (400g) of calcium carbonate are added to every sack of flour in this country, except 100 per cent wholemeal flour and self-raising flour. Wholemeal flour (which is naturally higher in calcium than white flour as well as in phytic acid) is exempted in recognition of those who want an 'unfiddled with' product. Self-raising flour is exempted because the baking powder used in it contains extra calcium anyway.

The practice led to the argument that wholemeal flour was, in this respect at least, bad for health. But it has since been established that people who eat wholemeal bread and/or oatmeal do not have any lower calcium status than anyone else. This seems to be because the digestive juices include an enzyme that can break down the calcium phosphate. This may be developed only when wholemeal products are eaten regularly – which would explain why the puppies Mallanby tested could not provide this enzyme. In addition, the phytic acid in wholemeal flour can be broken down by phytase in the flour itself, during the breadmaking process.

Oats contain very little phytase, but again, the digestive system can probably disarm the calcium-restricting action.

LOW CALCIUM INTAKES

Although calcium is still added to most flour, it is now done so not because of any fear of phytic acid, but because of the newer realization that hard water areas, with high water calcium levels, have lower heart disease rates than other areas.

The belief that the body can cope with phytic acid has strengthened with studies showing that some communities with low calcium intakes except from cereals do not suffer calcium deficiency.

The level of calcium absorption is also to some extent geared to the level of need. Children in communities where calcium intake is always low have been shown to develop normally on a total daily calcium intake of under 300mg. When the need of the bones is high, the absorption rate increases.

In a test on twenty-six Norwegian men, it was shown that twenty-two of them gradually adapted to a low calcium diet. This was measured by comparing the amount of calcium they ate with the amount they excreted each day. One of the men, for example, normally ate about 940mg of calcium a day, and he excreted about 840mg. So his body stores of calcium gradually built up. After nine months on a calcium level of just under 440mg per day, he was excreting only 320mg – but was still losing some calcium from the body. Eventually, he was excreting only 7mg of calcium a day, so that his body level was virtually in balance again.

About half of the men who adapted did so rapidly, and about half more slowly. But not everyone can cope with such a change: one man only adapted slightly, so he was losing a lot of calcium, and three did not adapt at all.

So quite a number of people cannot trust their bodies to absorb calcium more efficiently if supplies are reduced: they must make sure they get ample amounts. The more used we are to a high calcium diet, the less likely we are to be able to adapt our absorption to get enough from an unfamiliar low calcium diet. Older adults in any case absorb calcium less efficiently.

DEFICIENCY SYMPTOMS

Lack of calcium slows growth in children; in extreme cases, the result is rickets – common in British cities until the Second World War. Cities were affected more, it is thought, because children there also had poor access to sunlight that would have provided vitamin D to aid calcium absorption, and they often had poorer diets in general.

In older people, lack of calcium causes osteoporosis: brittle bones due to loss of calcium and protein. This makes them vulnerable to fractures. Osteoporosis is also caused by long-term use of some drugs, particularly steroid drugs such as cortisone, which cause calcium loss. The relationship between calcium status and hormones is thus close, and shows itself in women after the menopause, where the discontinuance of oestrogen production by the body goes hand in hand with an increase in osteoporosis.

Osteoporosis causes weakness and shrinking of bone mass. This is the feature of ageing that leads to people actually shrinking in height as they grow old, and to changes in bone formation such as 'dowager's hump'. Unfortunately, neither extra calcium nor extra oestrogen hormones has been shown to arrest osteoporosis linked to ageing. It is possible that shortage of vitamin D – due to lack of sunlight on the skin or to lack of vitamin D-rich foods – could be the key.

What does affect osteoporosis is exercise. As mentioned above, lack of physical activity causes increased calcium loss. Osteoporosis is best prevented by keeping active, by an adequate supply of calcium, vitamin D and good general nutrition.

Other symptoms of calcium deficiency are nervous spasms and cramps. These are related to calcium's function in sending messages along the muscle nerves. Facial twitching, weak-feeling muscles, cramp and other muscle-nerve symptoms are often signs of inadequate calcium.

HOW TO GET ENOUGH CALCIUM

The table on page 30 shows how much calcium there is in an average portion of common foods.

Food	Calcium (mg)
1 oz. (25g) hard cheese	230
1 oz. (25g) cottage cheese	23
¼ pt. (150ml) milk	170
5 oz. (150g) carton natural yogurt	250
1 oz. (25g) almonds	70
watercress	252
1 oz. (25g) dried figs	80
4 oz. (100g) baked or haricot beans	52
1 oz. (25g) wholemeal bread (1 small slice)	8
1 oz. (25g) oats (very large bowl of porridge)	16
1 oz. (25g) carrots, old	14
4 oz. (100g) sardines, canned in oil	624
1 tablespoonful black molasses ¼ oz./18g)	137
1 oz. (25g) sesame seeds	31
1 oz. (25g) kelp	306

Calcium is also contributed in much smaller amounts by other foods: fruit, root vegetables, meat and fish. But it is the major sources which you should make sure you get enough of to build up to your daily requirement of at least 800mg.

People who do not eat fish or dairy produce should ensure calcium supplies from almonds, sesame seeds, pulses and wholemeal cereals.

Because vitamin D is essential for calcium absorption, exposure to sunlight is important. Milk, cheese, eggs and oily fish are also sources of vitamin D.

Since the efficiency with which we absorb calcium tends to decrease with age, just when more calcium begins to be lost from the body, ensuring adequate supplies of this mineral becomes more, not less, important. Anyone over the age of forty should therefore aim to include calcium-rich foods on every shopping list.

CALCIUM SUPPLEMENTS

If for any reason this is difficult to do, or if other calcium-depleting circumstances apply, as outlined earlier, extra calcium may be taken.

Doctors regularly supply calcium supplements, often with vitamin D, for elderly people and those taking corticosteroid drugs, or recognized as suffering from osteoporosis.

Calcium supplements can also be bought over the counter at any chemist or health food shop. Calcium sold in health food stores offer a choice of forms: as plain calcium, or as bonemeal, where the calcium is in a natural context of other minerals. Calcium is also available in the natural context of dolomite, a calcium-magnesium carbonate found in limestone, which is sold powdered in tablets. Dolomite has the advantage of contributing other trace element minerals as well. A fourth form of calcium is the chelated form. This is designed to overcome the absorption problem, by preparing the calcium in a combination with protein substances. These prevent the calcium combining with other would-be mates – which would form insoluble compounds. Instead, the calcium is protected until it reaches the part of the intestine where it is to be absorbed, and is then able to pass through the intestinal wall more efficiently.

Because of the curious and little understood loss of calcium caused by lack of activity, regular exercise may be as valuable as diet in retaining good calcium levels. There may be benefit in taking calcium-rich foods or supplements at bedtime, since there is evidence that calcium loss is highest during the night.

THERAPEUTIC USES OF CALCIUM

Calcium is used to treat the following symptoms: cramps and muscle spasms; insomnia; nervousness; pain related to spinal or other bone injuries; menstrual cramps.

A therapeutic dose is just over a gram of calcium per day, usually split into three doses.

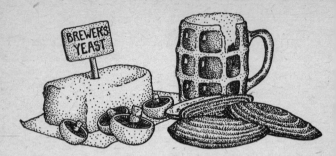

CHAPTER THREE

CHROMIUM AND COBALT

Only established as essential to man's health about ten years ago, chromium has blossomed into one of the most fascinating of trace elements. The fascination arises from the apparent link between the symptoms caused by lack of chromium deficiency, and two of the most rampant diseases of our time, diabetes and heart disease.

CHROMIUM AND DIABETES
The first evidence of chromium's vital role came from tests showing that rats on chromium-deficient diets lost their ability to maintain a healthy blood sugar level: they developed diabetic-like symptoms. They also had abnormally high levels of cholesterol in their blood, and were more likely to collect fatty deposits in the arteries of their hearts. There have since been many more tests confirming that chromium is necessary for man to deal with sugar in food.

It appears (for chromium's action is still little understood) that when sugar is eaten, and insulin is produced by the pancreas to enable it to be absorbed into the body from the blood-stream, chromium in the blood also increases. It comes from stores in the tissues, and probably works with the insulin.

Chromium is now considered part of a compound called the 'glucose tolerance factor', a substance known to be present in yeast, liver and kidney, which improves glucose tolerance in animals vulnerable in insulin disorders.

Several reports have claimed that giving extra chromium has a beneficial effect on diabetics. In one such test, four out of six patients with maturity-onset diabetes could deal with sugar better while being given 250 micrograms of extra chromium per day. In Jordan, Turkey and Nigeria, children who were poorly nourished grew faster if they were given extra chromium.

In the West, the implications are clear for diabetics and for those suffering from low blood sugar syndrome (where the body produces too much insulin in response to eating sugar, so that their level of energy falls abnormally fast and low after eating): eat more chromium, regularly.

CHROMIUM AND HEART DISEASE
The relationship between chromium and heart disease is even more interesting, since heart disease is what most of us die from.

There are three links. First, chromium-deficient rats who developed abnormally high cholesterol levels in their blood, and heart-clogging fat deposits; secondly, the fact that body levels of chromium are much lower in people in the West, who are so vulnerable to heart disease, than in those from the East, who rarely suffer from heart disease. People living in the Far East have been measured to have chromium stores several times higher than Americans tested. But if they emigrate to America, their offspring have lower chromium levels, and acquire the local vulnerability to heart attacks.

The third link between the metal and heart disease is that some reduction in cholesterol level has been achieved in some high-cholesterol patients by giving them chromium supplements. Only some patients improved, but this may be because the supplements given were not as sophisticated as they are today: chromium is one of those minerals which is extremely poorly absorbed, and hardly absorbed at all if given to the body in an unsuitable form. It's no use chewing up your car bumper!

INTAKE

Like most minerals, chromium is usually better absorbed by the body from food than from tablets. But even with food, the proportion absorbed may be as low as 3 per cent.

That means that how ever much we need in our bodies every day, we need many times more in the food we eat. No official body has yet set recommended daily intakes for chromium, and most estimates are based on measurements of how much is lost in urine. An adult loses about 7 to 12 micrograms a day. There is very little information either about how much the average person eats per day in food: one American reference gives itself a safe margin by estimating 5 and 100 micrograms! But with the known poor absorption rate, even the top figure might hardly be enough.

DEFICIENCY CIRCUMSTANCES

It is the digestion of sugar that calls on the body's insulin stores, so shortage is most likely to occur in people who eat a great deal of refined sugars, or whose ability to deal with sugar is already poor — such as diabetics.

It is interesting to note that natural sugars, in honey, blackstrap molasses, raw sugar and orange juice, for instance, all possess some chromium (see table below). White sugar, in contrast, has lost almost all the natural chromium which would have matched the chromium needed to digest the sugar.

Refined foods lose most of their chromium, so a diet based on these is likely to be deficient. White bread, for instance, contains less than a third of the chromium that was present in the whole wheat; the

Source	Average micrograms per gram
Glucose	0.03
White sugar	0.07
Dark raw sugar	0.24
Orange juice	0.13
Fructose or fruit sugar	0.18
Molasses, blackstrap	0.22
Maple syrup	0.18
Honey	0.29

Chromium in sweet things.

same applies to refined breakfast cereals, anything else made with flour, and white rice as compared to brown.

Pregnant women supply their babies with chromium. We have more chromium for our weight at birth than at any other time in life.

Slimmers who avoid high chromium foods such as wholegrain bread and cereals, nuts, meat and shellfish.

Chromium-deficient soils exist in some areas both naturally, and because of intensive farming with the same crop all the time. Crops grown on such soils cannot pick up chromium which is not there.

DEFICIENCY SYMPTOMS
No clear deficiency symptoms showing lack of chromium have yet been described, for long-term disorders of diabetes and heart disease are extremely difficult to pin to a single long-term cause, when we are subject to so many possible effects in life. One effect which has been linked with lack of chromium is an inability to tolerate alcohol – because of its rapid delivery of pure sugar to the bloodstream.

HOW TO GET ENOUGH CHROMIUM
By far the richest, best-established, simplest source of chromium is brewer's yeast. It is available in either tablet or powder form. No exact guidance can be

given on how much to take, but a few a day regularly would be sensible.

Present methods of measuring the chromium content in food are still slightly unsatisfactory, in that they do not show how much of the total chromium is in a form which the body can use. But the following foods are recognized as rich in usable chromium (in alphabetical order).

> Beef
> Beer
> Blackstrap molasses
> Brewer's yeast
> Grape juice
> Kidneys
> Liver
> Mushrooms
> Shellfish
> Wholewheat bread and cereals

COBALT

Evidence that cobalt was essential to nutrition first emerged in the 1930s. Investigations in Australia to identify the cause of wasting diseases in sheep and cattle showed that giving the animals cobalt or liver supplements cured the disease.

Later it was realized that the direct cause of the diseases was a deficiency of vitamin B12, which the animals were unable to produce because they lacked the cobalt necessary for that process. The soil the animals grazed was low in cobalt, so the grass and hay they ate was too.

In 1948, cobalt was discovered to be part of the vitamin B12 molecule. Unlike animals, humans cannot use the cobalt which also occurs separately from B12 in food to make their own B12 in the body: so the separate cobalt we eat may not matter. If we get enough vitamin B12, we get enough cobalt with it.

However, this does not explain why the body absorbs some of the separate cobalt in food (between 100 and 600 micrograms are thought to be eaten daily). This suggests that the body may need it for some other purpose, although no such purpose has been identified in man. In animals, cobalt has been reported to be required by the body to make thyroid hormone.

As part of vitamin B12, which is itself needed by the body only in very small amounts, our cobalt requirement is minute: it forms about 4 per cent of the vitamin, of which only about 10 micrograms per day are thought to be needed by adults.

DEFICIENCY CIRCUMSTANCES

As far as we know so far, a deficiency of cobalt means a deficiency of vitamin B12. This vitamin is vital to many body functions, including production of new tissue, red blood cells, bone marrow; growth; food metabolism; the health of the optic, nerve and mental systems.

Strict vegetarians or vegans are vulnerable to vitamin B12 deficiency, since the substance is almost exclusive to animal foods.

Failure to absorb vitamin B12 occurs in people who lack 'intrinsic factor', and the right stomach and intestinal acids. The result is pernicious anaemia, which can now be treated by injections of vitamin B12.

DEFICIENCY SYMPTOMS

No deficiency symptoms of cobalt, as a substance separate from vitamin B12, are known.

HOW TO GET ENOUGH

As explained above, getting enough vitamin B12 is by definition getting enough cobalt – as far as our present knowledge goes.

Cobalt supplements are not available, as there is no known benefit from taking them. Indeed, in spite of man's need for some cobalt, too much has been shown to be harmful. Too much cobalt would produce goitre by interfering with the thyroid gland. In 1966, heavy beer drinkers in some American cities suffered heart failure after drinking vast amounts of beer to which cobalt had been added to improve the appearance of the 'head'. But you cannot get an overdose of cobalt from food.

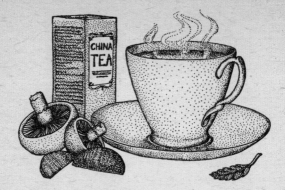

CHAPTER FOUR

COPPER AND FLUORIDE

The adult body contains between 100 and 150mg of copper, with the highest concentration in the liver. Copper's functions in the body are still poorly understood, although it is known to be part of several enzymes and proteins. What is not clear is whether it has a separate role, and acts directly.

What is clear is that without small amounts of copper, the body cannot form red blood cells. This was established in 1928, but finding out more about copper is taking a long time. Iron metabolism is dependent on copper, and deficiencies of either can cause a very similar anaemia in animals. Copper is necessary for enzymes needed for bone growth.

The concentration of copper in the body is highest at birth, perhaps as a reserve for the baby to use during its months on a milk diet (which is low in copper).

In animals, lack of copper (usually due to a high level in the soil of an antagonistic mineral, molybdenum) leads to diarrhoea, changes in the hair of the coat, and production of some fatty acids is reduced. The changes in animal hair caused by copper deficiency include both loss of hair, and loss of hair colour. No simple connection can be drawn between copper and loss of hair or greying in humans yet, but copper is thought to be involved in the formation of the pigment melanin.

Copper is also part of the production by the body of ribonucleic acids (RNA), the proteins that form the nucleus of every cell, and are the closest thing we know to being 'the building blocks of life'. RNA are also the carriers of genetic characteristics from one generation to the next. The copper requirement of an adult is probably between 1.5 and 2mg per day.

DEFICIENCY CIRCUMSTANCES

Newborn children can suffer from copper deficiency, particularly if they are premature, low weight or weaned too early on to cereals and cows' milk. In the first two cases, this is probably because the baby's body store of copper has not had the full time to build up; in the second, because refined cereals and cows' milk do not provide enough copper.

The copper in cows' milk may also be difficult for the baby to absorb, because this milk is high in zinc, a mineral which inhibits copper absorption by the body. Some babies may also be less efficient in building up a copper store.

Processed food fans get far less copper from food, since refining removes large amounts from wheat, rice, spaghetti, refined cereals and sugar.

Menke's syndrome is an inherited disorder which only affects boys. Sufferers cannot absorb copper across the placenta from their mothers during pregnancy. The resulting deficiency usually shows up when a baby is a few months old. The condition is also known as the 'steely hair syndrome' because one of the characteristics is the stubbly, stiff, colourless hair of the sufferer, which looks a little like steel wool. It was the resemblance between this characteristic and the fleece of copper-deficient sheep which led to Menke's syndrome being traced to lack of copper.

Other characteristics are more serious, including brain damage and seizures. Nowadays, babies may be given copper supplements as soon as they are born, but damage may already have occurred in the womb.

Some rheumatoid arthritis sufferers have a higher than normal level of copper in their blood. But this may mean that they are deficient in copper, or cannot retain it in their bodies. The copper in the blood is being taken from body stores, the theory argues, to compensate for lack of new copper being taken in.

Ill people may be unable to absorb copper normally.

Oral contraceptive takers have depressed blood levels of copper (along with a number of other nutrients).

Drugs such as penicillamine, which cause copper excretion, may lead to deficiency.

Pregnant mothers, passing copper to their babies, need extra.

Interference with absorption of copper can be caused by zinc, cadmium, fluorine and molybdenum, when they are present in high amounts compared to copper. Such interference has led to copper deficiencies in animals and occasionally in humans living in areas with unusually high soil levels of molybdenum and fluorine. Food and water in these areas then lack copper.

DEFICIENCY SYMPTOMS

There are few clearly recognized symptoms of copper deficiency in adults, except in communities living on subsistence diets. Loss of hair colour may sometimes be traceable to copper deficiency. So may loss of taste, which has been linked with deficiencies of copper and zinc, although no one yet understands how the mechanism is affected. In one study, about one third of drug patients being treated with penicillamine developed blunting of their sense of taste, which was restored when they were given copper supplements.

Raised blood cholesterol is caused in animals by a diet low in copper, and heart disease sufferers have been shown to have lowered levels of copper in the body.

Babies with copper deficiencies suffer from severe diarrhoea, fail to thrive and develop anaemia. They also fracture bones easily. Restoring copper clears up these symptoms, provided it is not left too late so that growth never catches up.

HOW TO GET ENOUGH COPPER

Given the low daily requirement, people who eat a varied and balanced diet should obtain enough from food.

High copper foods (at least 1mg of copper per 3½ oz./100g of the food).	Shellfish, yeast, liver, wheat germ, brazil nuts, malted products, cocoa, curry powder.
Medium copper foods (0.4-1.0mg of copper per 3½ oz./100g of the food).	Wholemeal bread, wholewheat cereals, mushrooms, parsley, broad beans, treacle, yeast and beef extract.
Some copper (0.1-0.4mg per 3½ oz./100g of the food).	Most meat and fish, pulses, nuts, dark green vegetables, red wine, cream.

Other foods are poor sources, particularly sugar, dairy products and refined cereals.

Copper supplements are available in the form of chelated copper (enclosed in protein form to improve absorption). These are used in cases of anaemia (to counter deficiency caused by taking medicines) and by some people to try to avert hair greying, although this effect is not established.

THERAPEUTIC USES OF COPPER

The often-mocked practice of wearing a copper bracelet for rheumatism and arthritis is on its way to becoming medically respectable. Copper may be absorbed through the skin, particularly where perspiration is present. Now copper has been shown to increase the anti-inflammatory powers of medicines, as well as being slightly anti-inflammatory itself.

Copper is used on some models of intra-uterine contraceptive devices (IUDs).

FLUORIDE

Fluoride has become almost a 'dirty word' in recent years, yet it and fluorine, the simple form of the mineral, are now almost established as an essential trace element.

Fluorine was first detected in animals by Gay-Lussac in 1805. But it is only recently that tiny amounts of fluorine have been shown to be necessary for normal growth in rats, and diets low in this element to result in lower fertility and anaemia in female mice.

Traces of fluorine are found in human tissues, especially in the thyroid gland, skin, teeth and bones. This does not of itself prove that fluorine is required by man, for it could be present as a pollutant. But there is increasing support for the belief that fluorine does have a use in the body of man, as it does in animals. This was strengthened in 1972 by a report that fluorine improved the density of bones in people suffering from osteoporosis (see Calcium, p.23).

It is also known that the body absorbs some fluoride out of food and drink, some of it being retained in the bones and in teeth which have not yet grown through the gum. More fluoride is retained during the fast growth period of childhood.

So far, we do not know any more details of what fluorine's role may be. The controversy over fluoride, the name used for fluorine as it occurs in food and drink, is not concerned with whether fluorine is necessary to man, but only whether dishing out more of it is beneficial or harmful.

The ability of fluoride to delay or arrest dental

decay in man was first noticed in the late 1930s. How it does this is not understood. It could be because it becomes part of the tooth enamel, making it more resistant to bacterial acid attack; or it might be that bacteria find fluoride such a hostile substance, they cannot grow in contact with it. Taking extra fluoride is no use to adults with fully developed teeth, which will not hold any fluoride.

FLUORIDE IN WATER

Meanwhile, every one gets some fluoride every day. Water is a far more important source than food, but the amount of fluoride in water varies widely from area to area. In Britain, water contains anything up to about six parts per million of fluoride. If you drink about $1\frac{1}{2}$ pt. (about a litre) of water (or a water-diluted drink) per day, you will get up to about 5mg of fluoride from it – depending on where you live.

The 'food' with the highest fluoride content is tea, especially China tea, and the tea-loving British obtain about 3mg of fluoride a day if they drink six strong cupsful.

Seafood is the only other significant food source, although many foods contain traces of fluoride.

The total daily intake is therefore very variable: non-tea drinkers in low fluoride areas receive virtually none, while other people in high fluoride areas may drink their way to an intake of about 8mg per day.

DEFICIENCY CIRCUMSTANCES

Children in low fluoride water areas may have worse tooth decay than high fluoride areas, but apart from this symptom, it is so far impossible to judge what the ideal intake of fluoride might be, or whether deficiency is possible or likely.

The proposed addition of fluoride to water supplies would mean an average person taking in 1mg extra of fluoride per day. If fluoride is only a few parts per million higher than that in water, it reaches the point where it gradually causes mottling on the teeth of those who drink it. The change in colour becomes more extreme and affects more people as the fluoride intake rises: white specks become brown stripey markings and teeth become rough and pitted. Mottling is not reversible.

The susceptibility of teeth to mottling varies considerably with the individual.

DEFICIENCY SYMPTOMS
Apart from possible tendency to more tooth decay, above, no deficiency signs are known.

HOW TO GET ENOUGH FLUORIDE
In the present situation, we can ignore our fluoride intake, unless we know that our local water content and tea-drinking habits add up to more than about 5mg per day. Every part per million of fluoride in our water contributes about 1mg of fluoride per day, if we drink about a litre of water (1¾ pt.) per day. Every cup of tea contributes about ⅓mg (from the tea alone); the stronger you brew the tea, the higher its fluoride content.

THERAPEUTIC USES OF FLUORIDE
Apart from the disputed therapeutic value of adding fluoride to water, none. The possible value of fluorine in helping avoid loss of bone strength with age is not yet established, while the ill-effects of even small overdoses of fluorine are.

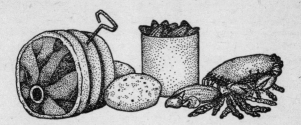

CHAPTER FIVE

IODINE AND IRON

Iodine was the second mineral – after iron – to be recognized as essential to man. The element was identified in seaweed in 1811, and in 1820, a Swiss doctor called Coindet successfully used iodine to treat sufferers from goitre – enlargement of the thyroid gland in the neck. By the end of the nineteenth century, it was known that the thyroid gland contained iodine, and that the enlargement was a direct result of lack of iodine, which makes the gland swell in an effort to extract more from the bloodstream. The adult thyroid gland contains about 8mg of iodine, out of a total of between 20 and 50mg in the body. The rest is in the hormones the gland produces.

Iodine is unique among the minerals: as far as we know, it is the only one which is an essential ingredient of particular hormones.

The thyroid hormones control the body's whole rate of activity. Insufficient hormone production leads to the whole system slowing down. Iodine is thus indirectly but closely connected with more than a hundred enzyme systems controlled by the thyroid hormones, including energy production, growth, reproduction, nerve function in the muscles, skin and hair growth.

There is no clear knowledge of how much iodine we need for health. The Department of Health and Social Security recommended a figure of 150 micrograms per day in 1969, but other bodies have suggested figures from 50 up to 300 micrograms per day.

DEFICIENCY CIRCUMSTANCES

In spite of the early realization of the curative use of iodine for goitre, this disorder is still suffered by about 6 per cent of the world's population (1960 figures), or about 200 million people.

The high rate of deficiency is because it is caused by geographical circumstances, so whole communities tend to be affected. The best source of iodine is seafood, which may not be available to people living inland. They therefore rely on meat, cereals, dairy foods and vegetables for iodine. But these foods can only supply the mineral if it is present in the soils where the crops are grown or the animals graze. Many parts of the world have iodine-deficient soils.

In Britain, hilly limestone areas such as Derbyshire and the Cotswolds are notably iodine-deficient, and goitre is also called 'Derbyshire neck'. Any areas where the rock is porous limestone is likely to be affected.

Not eating seafood regularly – at least twice a week – increases the chance of iodine deficiency. Boiling fish allows up to half the iodine to be lost in the water, and this should be avoided, or the water used in cooking. Recently, the possible iodine loss from frozen fish during thawing has been questioned, and this is being examined.

GOITROGENS

These are substances which prevent the thyroid gland extracting the iodine it needs from the bloodstream. Some goitrogens are known: high levels of cobalt and manganese, for instance, or a large intake of plants of the cabbage family can all interfere with iodine availability. This does not mean that cabbage is not a good food, but that like most foods, it should not be eaten *ad infinitum*, pounds and pounds of it every day. An outbreak of iodine deficiency in Tasmania, for example, was traced to milk produced by cows fed largely on brassica plants such as kale. The animals had eaten literally dozens of pounds of the vegetable, and the goitrogen had been concentrated in the milk. Tasmania is a region with little iodine in soil or water.

Other goitrogens are thought to exist but have not been clearly identified.

Pregnant and breast-feeding women are more vulnerable to iodine shortage because they pass on supplies to the growing child. Insufficient thyroid hormone leads to restriction of normal brain development in babies, and in extreme cases, leads to deaf mutism or cretinism.

Women are more vulnerable than men to iodine deficiency, and particularly so at times when their hormonal activity is changing, at puberty and during adolescence particularly.

High goitre areas have been shown to be areas with a higher than normal incidence of cancer of the womb – leading to a recent suggestion that women living in low iodine areas should make a positive effort to raise their intake of iodine-rich foods.

DEFICIENCY SYMPTOMS

Iodine deficiency leads to the following symptoms: enlarged thyroid gland, which can vary considerably in degree, but can be so extreme as to restrict breathing, and gives a clearly visible thickened neck; sluggishness in every area of life, physical and mental, with poor circulation and low vitality; dry skin, and a characteristic coarsening of the features caused by accumulation of material under the skin; dry hair.

HOW TO GET ENOUGH IODINE

Eating sea food is the surest way of obtaining iodine.
Two meals including sea fish a week should prevent
outright deficiency. The other iodine-rich seafood is
seaweed, including kelp, carrageen and laver bread.

Since cereals, meat and vegetables are all
unreliable sources, because their iodine content
depends on the soil of the area, the only other
certain sources are iodized salt, sea salt and fish liver
oils. Water is low in iodine – even sea water.

Iodine supplements are not sold as such, but kelp,
in powder and tablet form, is readily available in
health food stores. Carrageen 'moss', dulse and
Japanese seaweeds such as wakame and nori are all
reliable and available sources. Iodine deficiency is
very rare in Japan, where seaweeds are an everyday
food.

THERAPEUTIC USES OF IODINE

Once diagnosed by a doctor, iodine deficiency is
treated either with iodine itself or with thyroxine,
the iodine-containing hormone produced by the
thyroid gland.

IRON

Iron is the best known mineral, largely because so
many people have experience of being short of it –
and of taking extra iron to make up.

Of the total of about seven million pounds spent
by the National Health Service each year on vitamin
and mineral supplements, just under half is
expenditure on iron and other preparations that
encourage the formation of red blood cells.

Iron was the first mineral to have its main function
in man identified: by 1831, it was realized deficiency
of iron causes anaemia (although this is not the only
cause of anaemia). A healthy adult contains between
3 and 4g of iron. More than half of this amount is in
the form of haemoglobin, the red colour of blood.
But iron is also present in the tissues, and about a
gram is stored, mainly in the liver.

The iron is needed for two main jobs, although there may be others. Most of the iron used by the body is required by the bone marrow to make haemoglobin for new red blood corpuscles. As each corpuscle lives for about 120 days, approximately 1/120th of the total number must be replaced each day to maintain the right number. The other iron in the body is also renewed on a continuous basis. Some of the iron in the body is recycled, but the rest must come from outside. Once haemoglobin is formed, it carries oxygen in the blood from the lungs to the tissues, where other iron-containing substances use the oxygen.

The continual and adequate supply of oxygen is vital to every moment of life. Without enough iron, new red blood cells will be smaller and contain less haemoglobin – resulting in oxygen starvation all over the body. Our efficiency in every function is quickly affected.

PROBLEM OF ADEQUATE SUPPLY
Thus iron is one mineral whose vital nature has long been recognized. But the problem of adequate iron supply has not been solved. It is accepted that a large proportion of even affluent people suffer from iron deficiency in different degrees.

This is for three main reasons. First, people are not knowledgeable about which foods will provide them with iron – so they do not choose enough iron-rich foods.

Second, even when the food eaten contains a lot of iron, the body is very inefficient at absorbing it in the form in which it occurs in many foods. Generally, iron is much more efficiently absorbed from meat and fish than from foods of plant origin. Only 5 per cent or less of the iron in some foods may be available to the body, and 15 per cent absorption is about the maximum. The ability to absorb iron also varies with individuals, and within an individual, depending on other nutritional circumstances.

Only in recent years has the absorbability of the

different forms of iron in different foods been investigated. In 1972, for example, a study was published showing that the form of iron which for twenty years had been added to white flour, to try to make up for the loss in processing of the natural iron present in whole wheat, could barely be absorbed by the body at all. So a source of iron which had been counted on for a long time proved to be a complete illusion!

The third common cause of iron deficiency is that to make new, extra blood the body needs very high amounts of iron indeed – amounts difficult to supply from food. So women, who lose blood regularly, as well as in childbirth, are commonly iron-deficient. For the same reason, iron needs are very high during periods of growth, so that children's iron sources are extremely important. Women absorb iron about twice as efficiently as men – it has been estimated that 14 per cent of the iron in a non-vegetarian diet will be absorbed by women. But their needs can still easily outstrip the supply.

INTAKE

The official figures for recommended iron intake take these needs and absorption problems into account.

Recommended daily iron intake	Milligrams
Under 12 months	6
1 – 2 years	7
3 – 6 years	8
7 – 8 years	10
9 – 11 years	13
12 – 14 years	14
15 – 17 years	15
Men	10
Women up to 55	12
Women over 55	10
In pregnancy or breast-feeding	15

The figures are based on an estimated daily need

for *absorbed* iron of between ½ and 1mg, for an adult, so they count on about 10 per cent absorption. In fact it is estimated that the average daily intake of iron in the United Kingdom is about 12mg per day.

These figures might be satisfactory, if they did not assume a mixed diet when counting on 10 per cent absorption. For only the iron in meat and fish products is likely to be absorbed at or above that level.

Although the body can increase its absorption of iron to some extent when its needs for the mineral rise, the safety margin is narrow indeed, for such an all-important factor in well-being.

DEFICIENCY CIRCUMSTANCES

Women in their menstruating years are the most likely candidates for iron deficiency. Those who have heavy periods or who undergo blood loss in childbirth are especially vulnerable. Although women absorb iron more efficiently than men, anaemia is almost a commonplace with them, since few make an effort to ensure their iron supplies by wise food choice. The frequency of iron deficiency may be lower among women taking oral contraceptives, which usually reduce blood loss during menstruation; and higher among women using intra-uterine contraceptive devices, which usually increase blood loss in menstruation.

In pregnancy and during breast-feeding, iron in substantial amounts is transferred to the infant, drastically increasing the mother's requirements. Deficiency is likely to occur unless a deliberate effort is made to avoid it. Awareness of this problem has made iron supplementation almost automatic during pregnancy. But many woman do not take the supplements they are prescribed regularly. Either they do not realize their importance, or, very often, they find that taking the iron produces disagreeable indigestion and constipation, both already common during pregnancy.

Poor general diet clearly leads to iron deficiency by not making enough available. A tight budget does not mean a poor diet from an iron point of view, as several cheaper foods are actually richer in this mineral: sprats, liver, black pudding and sardines are all top iron suppliers! But sugar, fats and 'stodge' supply virtually no iron. Moreover, poor supplies of other nutrients will reduce the body's ability to use iron. Vitamin C enhances iron absorption, but a diet low in this vitamin will not help the body; copper, which tends to be lost in the processing of convenience foods, is an essential co-worker with iron. It both improves iron absorption, and its efficiency within the body.

Old people living alone are known, from careful studies, to neglect their general diet and often become iron-deficient.

Women on slimming diets can very easily become iron-deficient if they do not make a deliberate effort to include high iron foods in their programme.

Vegetarians do not eat the foods from which iron is most efficiently absorbed: meat and fish. So they would be vulnerable to deficiency were it not that most vegetarians are aware of this risk, and plan their iron supply. Soya beans, yeast extract and almonds are their best sources, and by eating substantial amounts of these and other vegetable foods relatively rich in iron, the vegetarian makes up for low absorption. In addition, a vegetarian diet is usually very high in vitamin C, and not so high in protein, both circumstances aiding absorption.

Convalescents from operations or any illness where blood is lost are candidates for iron deficiency, as new blood must be made just when both their food intake and absorption efficiency are likely to be lower than normal. Bleeding haemmorhoids, gastric bleeding due to ulcers, or to taking aspirins, will gradually deplete the body's iron status.

Fast-growing children are often iron-deficient, because of the body's unusually high requirement.

A low level of digestive acids diminishes iron absorption.

DEFICIENCY SYMPTOMS

Mild iron deficiency is often undetected, because its effects are so general. The first signs are lack of energy, susceptibility to infections and constant tiredness; but this gradual decline of health and *joie de vivre* as iron shortage builds up may be missed, or dismissed as being of emotional origin. Moreover, measurement of the iron level in the blood may not show up a borderline shortage, as the test only reflects iron in transit at a particular time, not the overall iron status of the body.

Severe iron deficiency does not happen suddenly, but develops over a period, as iron used fails to be replaced, using up the body stores. So it could be avoided if the earlier symptoms, above, were observed. After these, breathlessness, difficulty in swallowing and angina (pain caused by the heart muscle being starved of oxygen) develop.

Poor circulation can be another sign of lack of iron.

HOW TO GET ENOUGH IRON

The fact that iron is absorbed much more efficiently from animal foods has led to many nutritionists suggesting that these are the only good sources. The truth is that of the four top sources of iron in the British diet, three are vegetable foods: bread and cereals, potatoes and vegetables supply about two-thirds of our iron, while meat and fish supply about one-third. This is because we eat *more* of the vegetable sources. So vegetable sources are far from useless. But to ensure a good iron intake from vegetables, more must be eaten than one would suppose from looking at their iron content in food tables.

Many foods contain a little iron, but the following table shows which foods are important sources and classes them as 'high absorption rate', 'medium absorption rate' and 'low absorption rate'. These are shown by the letters H, M and L respectively. They represent approximate absorption levels of over 10, 10, 7 and 5 per cent of the level of iron shown in the table. These figures must be approximate, because of variations in iron content between samples and in absorption between individuals.

Keep in mind that the recommended daily intakes for an adult of 10mg for men and 12mg for women tend to be low. American figures are also 10mg of iron for men, but 18mg for women during their reproductive years. It is worth aiming for a really high intake from food, so that low absorption will not make you one of the thousands whose lives are less than lively through iron shortage.

Good iron sources	Mg/100g	Absorption
Black pudding and sausage	20	H
Liver	11	H
Kidney and heart	6	H
Game – hare, pheasant, pigeon, duck, etc.	3.5	H
Shellfish – oysters, cockles, winkles, whelks, mussels	7	H
Soya beans	2.5-3	M
Apricots, figs dried	4.1	L
Sardines	3	H
Corned beef	3	H
Beef, lamb	2-3	H
Molasses	16	L
Almonds, coconut	4	L
Pulses – lentils, peas, beans	1-2	L
Pumpkin, squash kernels	11	L
Prune juice, canned (no added sugar)	4	L
Oatmeal	4	L
Wholewheat bread	3	L
Wholewheat flour	4	L
Watercress, spinach and other leafy vegetables	1.5-3	L
Yeast extract, e.g. Marmite	7	M

Bran, brown rice and eggs look like reasonable sources, but the iron in them is thought to be very poorly absorbed.

As with most nutrition planning, it is not necessary

to think about iron supplies on a carefully counted, day-to-day basis. Getting enough iron is more a question of regularly including iron-rich foods on your shopping list or meal rota.

These foods should be given preference to the non-contributors: sugars, fats, cakes, sweets, soft drinks, ice cream, refined cereals and flour, sweet biscuits, and variants of these foods which give little iron (and usually little of other food elements too) for their calories.

The iron in vegetable foods like beans has been shown to be much more efficiently absorbed when some meat was eaten at the same time; this is attributed to an amino acid (protein) in meat called cysteine, which helps break down iron compounds into an absorbable form. Vitamin C substantially improves iron absorption, although figures are not available; so a salad/fruit/fruit juice serving in a meal will improve its iron contribution.

A rough and ready guide for people eating a mixed diet, is that men will absorb about 6 per cent and women about 8 per cent of the iron in food – so multiply the iron level stated in food tables by those figures to see whether you are getting at least the 1 and 2 mg a day that men and women are thought to need respectively to give a reasonable safety margin.

Cooking does not cause large iron losses from food, although vegetable cooking water contains some minerals, and should be used. Cooking can add to the iron in food if done in iron vessels, or using steel knives since iron can be leached from these into the food.

THERAPEUTIC USES OF IRON
Iron-rich diets are particularly valuable for post-operative convalescents; for women before and after childbirth and all during breast-feeding; for growing teenagers; for women who lose a lot of blood at menstruation; and for those taking aspirins or similar drugs to relieve arthritis, since aspirins cause gastric bleeding which can mount up with regular use. When food passes through the digestive

system abnormally fast, as in diarrhoea, less iron will be absorbed, and extra needed.

But trying to make up iron deficiencies by eating more iron-food may not always be practical, particularly in our calorie-conscious era. The iron in bread, for instance, is not only poorly absorbed, but increasingly uneaten as bread consumption declines.

Iron salts given by mouth are the normal medical answer, and these are usually given in very large amounts to offset poor absorption. Iron salts cause constipation or indigestion in some people, however, and many people prefer to take their iron in an organic form. This is the reason behind the popularity of iron-fortified tonics and tonic wines. Molasses and desiccated liver are both ways of taking extra iron in a non-bulky form. Many products based on these two items, and on iron derived from food, are available from health food shops. Chelated iron tablets, where the iron is put into a form that the body can absorb more effectively, are intended to overcome the absorption problem, which clearly causes as much iron deficiency as does lack of intake. They do not appear to cause the side-effects related to large doses of iron salts.

In recent years, it has been suggested by two independent studies that even when no anaemia can be detected, taking extra iron may improve resistance to fatigue and infection. Because of iron's interactions with other nutrients, however, tablets should always be seen as an addition to, not as a substitute for, a varied diet.

An interesting use for extra iron is the 'restless legs' problem. About one quarter of cases have been shown to be completely cured when iron supplements are given.

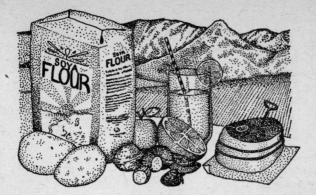

CHAPTER SIX

POTASSIUM AND SELENIUM

Our bodies contain a great deal of water: there are about 40 litres ($8\frac{1}{2}$ gallons, weighing $87\frac{1}{2}$ lbs) in someone weighing 65kg (approximately 143 lb). Five-eighths of this water are inside our cells; the rest is outside the cells. Maintaining this balance, and the correct composition of the cell fluids, is one of the basics of the body activity. Any disturbance in the mechanism causes fundamental and serious health problems.

Potassium is the main element in the water inside the cells, and sodium in the water outside the cells. So these two elements are crucially related in the fluid-balancing act. Every time we use a nerve or muscle, the pressure at the walls of the cells changes, and the result is that potassium is pushed out of the cell, and sodium enters. Then the original balance is restored. Most of our potassium is in our muscles, with an adult containing about 4 oz. (100g) of the element. A correct potassium balance is vital for nerves to react normally and for muscles to work properly.

Potassium also interacts with other elements,

taking part in such functions as converting glucose to muscle energy, enzyme reactions and the formation of protein. It also plays a vital role in the maintenance of the alkali-acid balance of the body (it maintains the alkalinity). No recommended daily intake for potassium has been set in Britain or in America, because of the wide variety of foods in which this element occurs. It is estimated that average potassium intake amounts to between 3 and 5g per day.

DEFICIENCY CIRCUMSTANCES

A high salt intake, which is the same as saying a high sodium intake, will encourage the kidneys to excrete more sodium in order to restore normal balance. In the process, more potassium will also be excreted, even if the body does not have any to spare. Today, most of us do have a high salt intake. This will be discussed under the heading of sodium (p.66), but it is an outstanding feature of modern eating patterns.

Diuretic medicines, taken daily by enormous numbers of people, are intended to reduce the body's fluid level. The use of these drugs has grown enormously in recent years in counteracting excess fluid present either as a result of high blood pressure or heart disease; or excess fluid retention caused by drugs such as cortisone, oral contraceptives, hormones, and others. These hinder the body's efforts to excrete sodium, which then holds water, leading to excess fluid in the tissues. Diuretics are also given frequently to women suffering from premenstrual tension, which is linked to excess fluid retention caused by hormonal swings at that time.

All diuretic drugs cause potassium loss along with the desired fluid loss. Although many brands (their names often including the letter 'K', the letter which is used to denote potassium) aim to restore the body's potassium level by including it in their ingredients, there is little to show that this prevents a net potassium loss.

Repeated use of anti-constipation medicines leads

to potassium loss, as the output of fluid from the body is increased. Diarrhoea from this or any other cause produces potassium loss.

Poor and processed food meals are often low in potassium, while contributing an overdose of sodium. Although potassium is present in very many foods, it is very low or absent in such foods as sugar, soft drinks, over-cooked vegetables, fats, white flour and white rice, spirits and, of course, everything made from these ingredients. Old people are especially vulnerable to failing to obtain enough potassium-rich foods.

DEFICIENCY SYMPTOMS

The first symptoms of potassium deficiency are weak muscles and mental confusion. A good deal of what appears to be loss of mental powers in old people can in fact be potassium deficiency showing itself.

Poor reflexes, constipation, nervous system disruption, a puffy abdomen and dry skin are other symptoms.

Severe deficiency leads to failure of heart muscle function – resulting in a heart attack.

HOW TO GET ENOUGH POTASSIUM

Although most natural foods contain potassium, some are far richer in the element than others. The amount of potassium in two samples of the same food can vary widely, but the following foods are rich sources: they are given roughly in descending order.

All kinds of dried fruit, especially prunes
Soya flour
Potatoes, especially unpeeled
Fresh fruit juices, especially citrus
Black treacle and molasses
Nuts
Bananas, prunes, apples
Instant coffee
Wholemeal flour and wheat germ

Conservatively cooked vegetables, especially
   leafy varieties
Meat
Fish

THERAPEUTIC USES OF POTASSIUM

Avoiding sodium-rich foods, and seeking out
potassium-rich ones instead, can be extremely
beneficial to anyone tending to retain excess fluid. A
day drinking only natural, unsweetened fruit juices
can produce dramatic losses of excess fluid in
women suffering from pre-menstrual tension or in
slimmers. However, dietary changes will not correct
the underlying disorder which causes fluid retention
in high blood-pressure, heart disease or when taking
certain drugs.

Potassium tablets of the chelated variety can be
bought in health food shops. A potassium salt is also
available for table use by people on low salt diets

Potassium supplements prescribed by doctors are
designed to correct established potassium
deficiencies: they are highly concentrated. These
tablets are liable to irritate the stomach, and may
encourage ulceration of the lining of the stomach or
intestine.

SELENIUM

Selenium's name comes from Selene, the Greek
name for the goddess of the moon. It has the special
property of conducting electricity when exposed to
light. This has made it extremely useful for technical
uses: it is essential to the design of Xerox machines,
for instance. It also has the unusual feature of being
distributed extremely unevenly in the earth's crust.

Selenium's importance to humans was only
established about twenty years ago. Because of its
variation from place to place, the same kind of food
grown in different areas can contain radically
different amounts of the mineral. So do different
water sources. This uneven distribution has meant
that some communities have high and some low
selenium supplies – a clearcut situation which has

helped studies trying to establish what the effects and functions of the mineral are.

For a long time, the only evidence about selenium was that high soil levels produced a kind of intoxication – 'the staggers' – in animals. Then it was seen that lower levels of selenium could prevent some of the symptoms of vitamin E deficiency in animals. Selenium and vitamin E are now always discussed together, and thought of as co-workers. Both act as anti-oxidants, i.e. they protect against the destructive effects of oxygen exposure on cells. Although the biological action of selenium is far from clear yet (the same enigma persists about vitamin E), this mineral has become one of the most talked-about and researched.

There have been studies comparing the disease rates in communities with high and low selenium levels in their blood. These seem to show that people living in high selenium areas have substantially lower rates of both cancer and heart disease. Selenium may in particular protect against breast and digestive tract cancers. This is a big 'may' so far. But in a study of mice who have been specially bred to develop breast tumours spontaneously, those mice who were given extra selenium had a much lower rate of cancer development.

SELENIUM AND HIGH BLOOD PRESSURE
Almost as dramatic are studies suggesting that selenium can in many cases among animals relieve high blood pressure, and, combined with vitamin E, the pain of angina in humans. In animals, selenium deficiency causes heart, liver and kidney failure. No wonder people are so excited about selenium. But the details of how it might work are still obscure.

OTHER FUNCTIONS
Selenium almost certainly plays a part in reproduction too. Selenium-deficient animals fail to reproduce; selenium is one of the ingredients of semen in men; half of a man's body selenium is concentrated in the testicles and the seminal glands

which are near the prostate gland.

It is known that selenium is part of an enzyme system, which controls the production of prostaglandins. These hormone-like substances in turn maintain many body functions, including some affecting the blood and blood vessel (and therefore circulatory) systems.

Selenium is thought to counteract cadmium, one of the 'bad' minerals known as heavy metals. Selenium's protective effect may be that it offsets the known health-destructive role of these heavy metals, which could be linked with cancer.

The idea that selenium and vitamin E both protect the body's cells from breakdown implies that they might be crucial to many functions – and in a few more years, we shall certainly have a much clearer idea of the details surrounding their action.

INTAKE

Meanwhile, it is not surprising that figures for how much selenium man needs are hard to find. In America a figure has been proposed – for a dog. It is 170 micrograms a day, for a body weight of 154 pounds or 11 stone – some dog. However, this is not a useful guide to deciding whether we get enough selenium, since there is no way for the average person to determine the selenium content of their food. If we lived on local food, we might be able to find out local selenium levels in the soil – but most of us eat food from many areas and countries.

This should actually reduce our vulnerability to a possible local selenium shortage.

DEFICIENCY CIRCUMSTANCES

Selenium is lost to some extent in food processing operations, with the largest losses being sustained during the milling of wheat to white flour and other cereals to their refined state. Cooking vegetables or other foods at high temperatures or for prolonged periods reduces their selenium content – although fruit and vegetables are not reliable sources in any case, thanks to soil variations and a relatively low selenium level to start with.

The diets of people who rely heavily on cereals and processed foods might therefore be low in selenium – but it is difficult to judge, because of the extremely wide possible variations. Smokers, who pick up large amounts of cadmium from tobacco smoke, may need larger amounts of selenium as their bodies use up the mineral to offset the cadmium's damaging effects. Other people may also be in contact wth large amounts of cadmium, mercury or arsenic (for instance from car exhausts for cadmium; from seafood for mercury; from seaweed or pesticide residues and accidental pollution of spices for arsenic). Smokers have this exposure in addition to the cadmium in tobacco smoke. Self-sufficient food producers living in very low selenium areas are at risk.

However, such theoretical circumstances have not been clearly identified as causing selenium deficiency symptoms in practice – at least, not yet.

It is thus extremely hard for the layman to identify deficiency. One symptom which has been linked with selenium deficiency is dandruff. Many people find a selenium-containing shampoo such as Selsun the only way to control dandruff. It may be that selenium shortage is related to this 'cause unknown' problem, but no firm link has yet been established.

HOW TO GET ENOUGH SELENIUM

Selenium sources that are less likely to be affected by geographical luck are seafood and meat. But the problem of selenium deficiency is so far too theoretical to make it worthwhile assuming you may have a shortage. A varied diet of unrefined foods should be the best defence.

THERAPEUTIC USES OF SELENIUM

Because of the toxicity of large amounts of selenium, no selenium supplements have been available until recently. Now a safe selenium supplement derived from yeast is available, in chelated form to aid absorption.

Selenium may be usefully taken in the amounts described on the product label when taking vitamin E – to enhance the vitamin's action. It *may* be helpful – and can safely be tried – in cases of dandruff, deteriorating eyesight, infertility or lost sexual ability; arthritis; for angina and for smokers. It is a mark of this mineral's elusive yet important character that its possible uses are at once so wide and so uncertain.

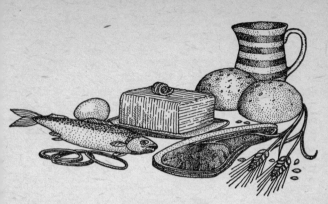

CHAPTER SEVEN

SILICON, SODIUM, STRONTIUM AND SULPHUR

SILICON

It's amazing to learn that this seldom-heard-of mineral makes up over a quarter of the earth's crust. Silicon is not yet firmly established as being necessary for man, although it is known to be so for other animals. So far, evidence of the role of silicon in man is limited to reports that silicon is present and may be important to the connective tissue between joints and organs; and that silicon as well as calcium plays a part in bone formation in young animals. Giving silicon to rats and chicks on low-silicon diets improves growth by 25 to 50 per cent. It has also been noted that the silicon levels in one of the heart vessels – the aorta – of rats, chicks and rabbits drop greatly when the animals age.

The use of silicon as a food additive makes it unlikely that any human need for the trace element is unmet. Silicon compounds are used to stop foods caking together, to help them run freely, or to prevent them from foaming unduly. Excess intake of silicon from the air in certain environments such as mines and quarries is the cause of silicosis, an extremely dangerous and often fatal occupational disease of workers in such areas.

DEFICIENCY CIRCUMSTANCES AND SYMPTOMS
None known in man. In chicks, stunted growth, abnormalities of bone formation, and atrophy of the organs result.

THERAPEUTIC USES OF SILICON
None known.

SOURCES OF SILICON
Unrefined cereals are the best source, with little of the element in animal foods. Beer consists of a saturated solution of silicon.

SODIUM
Sodium, with potassium, regulates the body's water transport balance in and outside cells. This is the mineral's basic function, and the average adult contains between 3 and 3½ oz. (75-87g) of sodium. Most of our body sodium is in our blood and the fluids around cells, while a substantial amount is built into our bones.

Although sodium is thus a vital mineral, and even relatively small losses – 10g or so – will cause severe deficiency symptoms, we suffer more from sodium excess than sodium deficiency. The amount of salt, which is pure sodium chloride, that we add to our food is far beyond our bodies' needs, and has bad effects in many cases.

INTAKE, SOURCES AND DEFICIENCIES
Although intake varies widely, most people probably take in about ten to fifteen times as much sodium as they need each day. Indeed, we do not need any added sodium from salt in our diets – there is enough in natural foods.

Almost every prepared food has salt added to it: bread has about a hundred times more sodium than wheat; butter, bacon, cheese, corned and pickled meat, sausages and salami, margarine, tinned fish, even breakfast cereals are all high in sodium, while their untreated raw materials are not.

Sodium deficiency is possible in hot climates, or following strenuous physical exercise in hot weather. But for most purposes, sodium belongs with the minerals we get too much of – and is discussed further in that chapter (p.85).

STRONTIUM

Firmly connected in most of our minds with strontium 90 – the radio-active form of the mineral which is a by-product of nuclear bombs – strontium is also a standard element of our bodies and environment.

Discovered at the end of the eighteenth century, strontium behaves in many ways like calcium. It is stored in the bones, and is found in the same foods which supply calcium.

Little is known of its functions, so far, or of how much the body may use.

DEFICIENCY CIRCUMSTANCES
None known.

DEFICIENCY SYMPTOMS
None known.

SOURCES OF STRONTIUM
Dairy foods, and fresh vegetables.

THERAPEUTIC USES
None known.

SULPHUR

Animals and plants all contain protein, and all proteins contain some sulphur. So this element is both essential and closely linked with protein. The element forms an ingredient of several essential protein substances of B vitamins thiamin (B1) and biotin, and of other compounds inside the body.

In this way, sulphur is needed if many functions are to take place correctly. Yet the way in which sulphur forms compounds and the amounts involved is not clear. Although sulphur is present in every cell, it is concentrated in hair, nails and skin. An adult contains about 4 oz. (100g) of sulphur.

Protein foods are the richest sources of sulphur although vegetable foods supply some too. Because this element is so widespread in food, there is no likelihood of deficiency, and no recommended figure for daily intake. However, 850mg a day is thought to be the required amount by American mineral researcher Carl Pfeiffer.

THERAPEUTIC USES OF SULPHUR
Sulphur has an old reputation as a blood cleanser, to be consumed in the form of brimstone and treacle. This was mainly to use the laxative properties of large amounts of sulphur to achieve a 'spring clean'. But any overpowerful laxative is only effective because the body is working its hardest to expel an unwanted excess. Sulphur is more useful as an external or oral treatment for skin complaints such as psoriasis, eczema and dermatitis – and is intimately linked with zinc and possibly selenium in maintaining the health of the skin, nails and hair.

DEFICIENCY CIRCUMSTANCES
Protein deficiency would involve sulphur deficiency.

DEFICIENCY SYMPTOMS
None established.

SOURCES OF SULPHUR
Rich sources are eggs, meat, fish, pulses and nuts; cabbages, onions and other greens contribute some too.

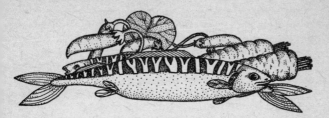

CHAPTER EIGHT

TIN, VANADIUM AND ZINC

TIN

Still not to be found in many discussions of minerals in human nutrition, tin is just on the borderline of acceptance as a necessary mineral for man. It has been more or less established as necessary for rats since the 1960s. Its functions, however, are so far quite unknown, as is how much we either contain or need.

However much our requirement for tin is, we almost certainly exceed it in our intake, thanks to tin transferred to food from the linings of tins and from cooking foil. Intake from these sources is estimated to range between 1 and 4mg per day.

Tin linings in food cans dissolve quickly in contact with oxygen in the air. This is why food should not be stored in opened tins. Legally, food is not permitted to contain more than 250 parts per million of tin. However, this ruling is broken in many cases, where acidic foods are able to leach tin from the linings of cans. How harmful this might be is not well established.

DEFICIENCY CIRCUMSTANCES AND SYMPTOMS
None known.

THERAPEUTIC EFFECTS OF TIN
None known.

VANADIUM
The belief that vanadium is essential to man is recent, and grows out of our knowledge of its importance to several kinds of animals. Deficiency symptoms can be produced in several species by giving food lacking this element.

The results for rats, for example, are retardation of growth, shortened lifespan, poor reproduction and an abnormally high level of cholesterol in the blood. Chickens kept short of vanadium also show high blood fat levels – and this characteristic of vanadium is enough to make the element intensely interesting to our heart disease-ridden age.

Tests to see whether vanadium can bring down cholesterol levels in human blood have had mixed results. Some people who took the extra vanadium had lowered levels but the amount required to achieve this was higher than could normally be obtained from food – suggesting that it is not a lack of a normal amount of the element in food that causes raised blood cholesterol levels.

Nevertheless, the two features may be related and vanadium clearly has the ability to slow up the body's own production of cholesterol. There is no estimate of human requirement for vanadium.

DEFICIENCY CIRCUMSTANCES
Limited tastes in food could lead to low vanadium intake, as meat, milk and vegetables are all poor sources.

Processing which can cause loss of minerals could reduce the amount available to the eater.

DEFICIENCY SYMPTOMS
None established yet in man.

HOW TO GET ENOUGH VANADIUM
Unrefined cereals, nuts and root vegetables are the best sources – no one knows how much is required.

THERAPEUTIC USES

None as yet known.

ZINC

Partly thanks to its association with sexual development, zinc has enjoyed an enormous amount of attention from both researchers and journalists in recent years. Its functions in life processes was first observed in 1869, when a biologist noticed that a plant would not grow when zinc was absent. Zinc has since been established as necessary for the normal growth of plants and animals, including man.

Full recognition of its importance had to wait until the invention of techniques for analyzing its presence in hair or blood in the 1950s. The existence of people with severe zinc deficiency in Iran and Egypt was then revealed, showing dwarfism, lack of sexual development, poor hair growth and rough skin. The deficiency was the cumulative result of low levels of zinc in the local water, poor diet and in some cases, poor absorption. Giving extra zinc produced marked improvements. The mechanism by which zinc acts is still not completely understood, but is related to the fact that zinc is an essential ingredient of many enzymes.

There is no recommended daily intake, but adults are estimated to need between 15 and 20mg of zinc a day. The mineral is particularly crucial during pregnancy, as even temporary deficiency could lead to abnormalities in the offspring, and during growth, which lack of zinc will hinder.

DEFICIENCY CIRCUMSTANCES

Zinc deficiencies are probably widespread, but not in such an extreme form that they are readily detected.

Poor absorption of zinc is common, and could cause shortages in those where general ability to absorb nutrients is below par. Old people and convalescents are at risk.

An excess of phytic acid, which is high in the outer

husks of cereals such as bran, reduces zinc absorption by combining with the element to form an insoluble compound. Phytic acid is broken down in the bread-making process, and people accustomed to wholemeal bread are thought to develop an enzyme capable of breaking down the phytate compound. However, the current fashion for 'bran with everything' could produce some zinc shortages. These could be avoided simply by eating bran in wholemeal flour, rather than as an isolated element.

Non-breast fed infants sometimes develop a formerly fatal condition known as acrodermatitis enteropathica. Although inherited, this illness, where there are lesions in the skin and chronic diarrhoea, is relieved by zinc supplements, which need to be taken permanently. The cause of the disease is thought to be that in the vulnerable baby, any protein except human milk protein combines with zinc and prevents its absorption.

Diabetics have abnormally low body zinc levels, and zinc is involved in the storage and release of insulin.

Heavy drinkers have low zinc levels, since alcohol depresses the mineral.

Processed food diets can lead to zinc deficiency, as the mineral is absent from fat, sugar and white bread.

Several drugs, including oral contraceptives lower body zinc levels. This is because they raise oestrogen levels, which produce low zinc in the blood.

Copper piping carrying water which is then drunk could depress zinc levels, as copper is antagonistic to zinc.

DEFICIENCY SYMPTOMS
Poor healing is well established as a zinc deficiency effect.

White spots or bands on the nails could be due to zinc deficiency, the mechanism being that the zinc binds to the protein albumen, the lack of this then causing white spots. Taking extra zinc will not remove large white spots, which have to grow out, but it should prevent recurrence of the effect.

Deteriorating ability to taste is a recently established effect of zinc shortage. Known as dysgeusia or hypogeusia, the sufferer may suddenly lose his ability to distinguish foods after an acute respiratory illness such as bronchitis; or may notice only a gradual diminution of sense of taste and/or smell. Such people have low body zinc levels, and respond well to supplements. The lack of sense of taste is accompanied by, or may be the cause of, loss of appetite. This in turn leads to reduced food consumption and weight loss.

In the four years since this effect of zinc deficiency was discovered, there has been interest in manipulating zinc intake as a method of tackling obesity. By giving an amino acid (protein) called L-histidine, zinc is removed from the system, and a controlled state of lack of appetite results. In studies conducted by Dr Robert I. Hinken, Director of the Centre for Molecular Nutrition and Sensory Disorders at Georgetown University Medical Centre, Washington, a group of young college students (not obese) who took extra L-histidine started eating less within a week, and losing two to three pounds a week as a result. Work is now in process to find the minimum dose of the protein which would achieve the desired effect, without causing any more undesirable symptoms of zinc deficiency than necessary. When the desired weight was achieved, extra zinc would rapidly restore both sense of taste and appetite.

No one should attempt to reduce their zinc intake from food on their own, in order to depress their appetite in this way. For most people, overall reduction in food intake is a new habit which should be worked at – spoiling appetite by reducing zinc would have to be continued lifelong if weight were not to be put on again. Such prolonged treatment might well be dangerous to general health.

On the other hand, people who are trying to slim would be wise not to take extra zinc.

HOW TO GET ENOUGH ZINC

The best food source of zinc is seafood, such as herring and oysters. Meat is the second richest source, while whole grains, nuts, peas and beans also contribute important amounts. Zinc tablets, in a chelated form for more efficient absorption, are sold over the counter at health food shops.

THERAPEUTIC USES OF ZINC

Zinc may be taken by people who also take drugs, in order to redress the drug-caused deficiency. Again influenced by oestrogen, zinc levels are very low in the week before a period, and restoring these may be beneficial.

Women planning a pregnancy should ensure that their food contains good sources of zinc, before and during pregnancy and breast-feeding. This will reduce risks of zinc shortage for the baby. Breast milk itself contains high levels of zinc for the first two weeks – ten parts per million – when this drops sharply to only a twentieth of that amount.

Convalescents from wounds or burns would be wise to ensure good zinc supplies in food or supplement form.

One of the most exciting and newest uses of zinc is to treat acne. After centuries of the use of zinc oxide in calamine, zinc taken by mouth has now been shown to have a substantial effect in reducing the number of eruptions. This has been attributed to zinc stimulating the formation of prostaglandins, hormone-like substances, and a lack of these being a cause of acne. A hormone-related cause for acne is likely, in view of the complaint's close correlation with times of hormone changes, such as puberty, menstruation and pregnancy.

What about zinc's link with sex? Although the mineral is certainly linked with normal sexual development during childhood, and possibly with fertility in men, there is no evidence that extra zinc, above normal amounts, will have an effect in increasing or enhancing sexual performance.

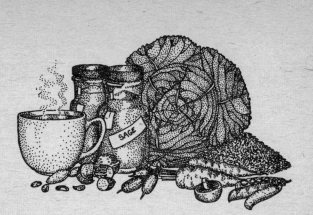

CHAPTER NINE

MANGANESE AND MAGNESIUM

MANGANESE

Manganese is one of the still mysterious trace elements whose main functions appear to be to 'trigger off' vital reactions. These cannot take place unless the trace element is present, yet it may not be actually involved once the process has started.

Processes for which manganese is thought to be necessary include structure-building of the young in the womb, growth, successful childbearing, the health of the nervous system, and the building of the proteins known as nucleic acids, which carry genetic information from one generation to the next.

As with many micronutrients, more of our knowledge is based on observation of what happens when there is a manganese deficiency than on understanding of how the element works inside us. A healthy adult is known to contain 12 to 20mg of manganese.

Two interesting associations with manganese have been shown. One study has shown that the manganese level in the blood of diabetics was approximately half as high as in a similar group of non-diabetics; and two studies have suggested that manganese can be useful in treating schizophrenia. Its supporters for this use point out that schizophrenics have abnormally high body levels of copper; and that manganese can displace copper from the body.

Neither Britain nor America has a recommended daily intake of manganese. It has been estimated that an adult excretes 4mg of the mineral a day, suggesting that a similar amount needs to be taken in daily. The daily intake in Britain is thought to be one to 20mg per day – a very wide variation.The absorbability of manganese from food has not been studied.

DEFICIENCY CIRCUMSTANCES
No clear case of manganese deficiency has been described in man, apart from the association with diabetics. Manganese-deficient soils have produced manganese deficiency in animals, since the grazing and crops were also short of the mineral. Peaty soils are the most likely to suffer. The deficiency symptoms we know of come from such places.

DEFICIENCY SYMPTOMS
In animals, deficiency results in poor growth and reproduction, with infertility and stillbirths; defects in bone formation and the nervous system in the infant, and anaemia. A single case of manganese deficiency in a man produced loss of weight, changes in hair colour, temporary dermatitis, attacks of nausea and a very low cholesterol level.

HOW TO GET ENOUGH MANGANESE
It is not surprising that manganese deficiency is unknown in Britain: an outstandingly rich source is tea! One cupful may provide 1mg of manganese. The other rich sources are nuts, spices, wholegrain cereals and dark leafy vegetables such as spinach.

However, when grains are refined, they lose most of their manganese, which is concentrated in the germ and bran portions which are removed from the white version. White flour has lost about 90 per cent of its manganese; white rice about 26 per cent.

So tea appears to be the only manganese-redeeming factor for those who eat refined carbohydrates, and who eat little of either nuts or green vegetables. Although spices are extremely rich, ounce for ounce, the tiny quantities of them which we eat restrict their contribution.

THERAPEUTIC USES OF MANGANESE

Some American practitioners using nutrient therapy for schizophrenics give manganese to lower abnormally high copper levels.

Because manganese is involved in the body's ability to cope with fats and glucose, manganese may help those with vulnerability to heart disease or to diabetes.

MAGNESIUM

All human cells contain some magnesium, adding up to a total of about 25g in the body of a healthy adult. About 60 per cent of this amount is in the bones, where it is probably in storage, to be called on if a shortage occurs elsewhere in the body.

Magnesium is one of the 'trigger' minerals: it is necessary to set off various body reactions, and together with calcium and potassium, it plays an important part in maintaining the balance of the cells. But, so far, the exact process in that role is unknown. Our knowledge abut magnesium is mainly of symptoms caused by lack of it.

Outright deficiency is thought to be rare in affluent societies. However, interest in magnesium has risen as a result of studies showing that people who had died from heart attacks had less magnesium in their heart muscle than people who died from other causes. Put together with the fact that deaths from heart disease are lower in areas with hard water (including more magnesium), this has led to the suggestion that higher magnesium intakes might be a wise step for the prevention of heart disease. But the theory is far from proved, since the low magnesium might be the result rather than the cause of the heart disease.

Due to this lack of evidence, there is no British recommended daily intake figure. In America, one has been set at 350mg per day for men, 300mg for women, rising to 450mg during pregnancy and breast-feeding. British people are estimated to obtain between 200 and 400mg of magnesium daily from food – a somewhat vague figure. Nor do we know how much of the magnesium we eat in food is absorbed – one estimate is about a third.

DEFICIENCY CIRCUMSTANCES

Poor absorption can be caused by prolonged diarrhoea, illness, and diuretic drugs (which make the body excrete extra fluid). Heavy drinking also causes loss of magnesium.

Convenience food eating reduces the level of magnesium in the diet, since the typical ingredients of such foods – a high level of fat, sugar, white flour, refined cereals, and soft drinks – contribute barely any of this mineral. Wholemeal flour contains up to five times as much magnesium as white flour; polishing rice to make it white removes five-sixths of the magnesium; refined maize, as used in cornflakes and cornflour, has lost three-fifths of this mineral.

DEFICIENCY SYMPTOMS

The first symptoms of magnesium deficiency are apathy, muscular weakness, depression, vertigo and over-excitability of the nervous system which controls the muscles – i.e., spasms or cramps. More serious deficiencies result in convulsions produced by the nerve-muscle system.

The close link between magnesium, potassium and calcium means that the body's balance of the two latter minerals is also upset by magnesium shortage. Indeed, magnesium deficiency symptoms were not identified as such for a long time because they overlapped with those known to be related to the two other minerals.

In studies of animals, lack of magnesium has been

shown to restrict the growth of new tissue and the body's use of protein.

HOW TO GET ENOUGH MAGNESIUM

Magnesium is an essential part of chlorophyll – so plant foods are rich sources, and vegetables and cereals are estimated to contribute about 70 per cent of the daily intake. However, most unrefined foods contain some magnesium.

Rich magnesium sources	mg/100
Seafood	
Wheat germ*	310
Almonds,* cashews*	270
Brazil nuts*	225
Soya beans	200+
Bran*	490
Wholemeal bread and crispbread	80
Green leafy vegetables	70–100
Apricots (dried)	62
Peanuts,* sesame seeds*	175
Walnuts*	130

Careless cooking of vegetables in too much water or for too long causes over half the magnesium to be transferred from the food to the water. This loss should be avoided, but in any case, vegetable cooking water should be used if possible in soup or sauce-making.

THERAPEUTIC USES OF MAGNESIUM

The balance between calcium and magnesium is important and should be preserved when thinking about supplements. Unless magnesium is known to be lacking, it is better to take both minerals together. The usual ration is to take twice as much calcium as magnesium.

Like calcium, magnesium is a nerve-soother, but in

* The phytic acid in these foods may to some extent reduce the magnesium available from them by combining with it to form an unbreakable compound which passes right through the body.

the physical rather than the psychological sense. Since a lack of it may lead to cramps, twitches, tremors, menstrual cramps and muscle spasms, taking extra magnesium may be the key to solving these problems.

In the same way, known magnesium deficiency symptoms, such as 'nerves', depression and apathy, encourage people who have no organic disease, yet suffer from such symptoms, to try magnesium to relieve them.

Some people living in soft water areas, low in calcium and in magnesium, take supplements to offset any increased risk of heart disease.

Extra magnesium is available in various forms. It is included in some multi-vitamin and mineral preparations. Or you can buy chelated magnesium tablets at health food shops. To obtain both calcium and magnesium, you can also choose the multi-vitamin type of preparation, or buy magnesium and calcium tablets separately.

Alternatively, dolomite, a naturally occurring combination of magnesium and calcium, is available in both regular and chelated forms, the chelated being designed to overcome poor absorption. Bonemeal tablets are another way of combining both minerals.

Laxatives and antacids which are based on magnesium salts – such as Epsom salts – are not the way to take extra magnesium. Their laxative effect drains valuable minerals, especially potassium, out of the body.

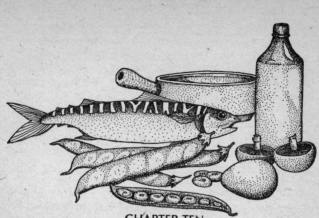

CHAPTER TEN

MOLYBDENUM, NICKEL AND PHOSPHORUS

MOLYBDENUM

The recognition of this metal as an essential trace element for man is based on its known presence in several enzyme systems. Little detail of its function is known, however.

One of the enzyme systems, known as xanthine oxidase, may be involved in the body's method of obtaining iron from certain iron compounds. So a deficiency of molybdenum might interfere with the body's iron supplies.

The same enzyme system is known to be involved in the breakdown of certain proteins to uric acid. This is a normal and necessary process; however, excess uric acid production leads to gout, the formation of uric acid stones in the urinary passage and increased vulnerability to heart disease. The only known link between this situation and molybdenum is a community in Armenia, whose uncommonly high rate of gout has been traced to unusually high molybdenum levels in the local soil.

This community's daily intake is estimated at 10-15mg a day, which has thus been established as an excess. But we do not know what an ideal intake would be; measurements of intake and body content taken in different places vary enormously, showing how much supplies of this mineral depend on soil content. Consumption of $\frac{1}{2}$ to 2mg per day has been considered normal.

DEFICIENCY CIRCUMSTANCES
Acid, sandy soils produce crops low in molybdenum High copper levels in soil or diet are antagonistic to molybdenum, and vice versa.

DEFICIENCY SYMPTOMS
None recognized, except that children in areas with high molybdenum levels in the soil have been reported to have fewer holes in their teeth than children from low molybdenum areas. This anti-tooth decay effect has been shown in animals.

HOW TO GET ENOUGH MOLYBDENUM
We cannot plan our molybdenum supplies for three reasons. First, we don't know how much to aim for. Second, the amount in the same food, but grown in different areas, will vary enormously. Third, the element is hard to measure.

THERAPEUTIC USE OF MOLYBDENUM
None known.

NICKEL
Not directly proved to be essential to man, nickel has only recently appeared in discussions on mineral nutrition. Interest in it has increased both because of the discovery of its presence in human tissue, and because it has been shown to be necessary to rats, pigs and chicks.

There is little evidence as to what role nickel may play in humans. People who suffer heart attacks may have an abnormally high level of nickel in their blood. Both existing and desirable levels of nickel are unknown.

DEFICIENCY CIRCUMSTANCES

None known. Deficiencies have been produced in test animals by altering their diet, but only with difficulty

DEFICIENCY SYMPTOMS

None known in humans. In animals, nickel seems to be needed for the healthy functioning of the liver. Poor growth of offspring, and liver malfunction have been seen.

HOW TO GET ENOUGH NICKEL

Whatever our requirement for nickel, modern man almost certainly acquires it ... and more. Nickel in tiny amounts is transferred from the alloys used to line saucepans; from food processing machines; from margarine, where nickel is involved in the hardening of oils, (and from cigarettes and cigarette smoke!).

THERAPEUTIC USES OF NICKEL

None known.

PHOSPHORUS

Phosphorus is closely linked with calcium in its functions and supply mechanism. It is second only to calcium in the amount we hold in our body: an adult contains from $1\frac{1}{2}$ to 2 lb (600-900g) of phosphorus. As with calcium, most of this is in the bones – that is, up to 85 per cent of the total.

The development and hardness of bones and teeth cannot take place normally without sufficient phosphorus. But the mineral also plays a vital part in the body's ability to turn food into energy. A third important function is as a constituent of nucleic acids, the proteins that carry inherited characteristics to the next generation.

There are no recommended intake figures for phosphorus in Britain because the mineral is so abundant in foods that no shortage is thought possible. The actual intake is thought to be about 1500mg per day. American suggested daily intakes are as follows:

Age	Phosphorus (mg)
Up to 6 months	240
6 months – 1 year	400
1 – 10	800
11 – 18	1200
Adults	800
Women during pregnancy or breast-feeding	1200

DEFICIENCY CIRCUMSTANCES

Antacids (indigestion medicines) combine with the phosphorus in food, making it unavailable to the body. Repeated use of these mixtures will lead to deficiency. Otherwise, deficiency is virtually unknown under normal circumstances.

DEFICIENCY SYMPTOMS

When not enough phosphorus is available from food, the body will take the mineral from the bones for use elsewhere. The result is weakening of the bones and lack of growth in children. Weaker bones are painful, particularly when carrying the body's weight.

HOW TO GET ENOUGH PHOSPHORUS

Phosphorus is present in almost all foods, and there is no need to make an effort to obtain it. The richest sources are the same as for calcium – dairy produce, meat, fish and eggs.

In addition to naturally-occurring phosphorus, we eat extra which is added by food processors. Baking powders, phosphoric acid in soft drinks, polyphosphates which reduce 'drip' and hold water in hams and frozen chickens, and emulsifying salts in foods like processed cheese add about 10 per cent to our total phosphorus intake.

THERAPEUTIC USES OF PHOSPHORUS

None. Phosphorus supplements, in any case, would upset the calcium-phosphorus balance, increasing the body's needs for calcium, a far less abundant mineral.

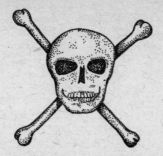

CHAPTER ELEVEN

MINERAL OVERDOSES

Minerals which can harm us can be divided into two groups. First are those essential elements which we need, but which will cause ill-effects if taken in excess. Second, there are some minerals for which the body has no use, and which can only harm us.

TOO MUCH OF A GOOD THING
An excess of a useful mineral can arise in several ways. Human error can dump a large amount of an element on us unseen – via animal feed, for example. Human bad habits can do the same – which is the present situation with sodium, piled on our systems by the general salt-with-everything practice.

In a very few cases, Mother Nature herself can be the culprit, distributing minerals so unevenly upon the soil that certain areas have excesses of some element or other.

Taking mineral supplements is very unlikely to result in trouble, unless the taker ignores the instructions on the bottle, and deliberately takes a large overdose. Minerals which would cause ill-effects even in small extra amounts – such as iodine –

are not sold as supplements except for prescription use. This chapter excludes deliberate overdoses, and discusses only excesses which could arise in normal life. And no one need worry about getting too much of a useful mineral from natural foods; in that context, they are amply diluted so that taking too much is impossible – without a deliberate and neurotic effort. Many ill-effects which could arise from over-consumption of a useful mineral are not the result of that amount proving harmful, but to its depressing the body's access to another element, causing symptoms of imbalance.

There could also be a long-term snag to taking regular and substantial supplements of useful minerals. In many cases, the body learns to absorb and use more of the mineral when it is in short supply; and lets more be excreted when the element abounds in the diet. So if we consistently eat a very high level of calcium, for example, we might be more vulnerable to calcium deficiency symptoms if our intake suddenly diminished, even if it were still at a level on which habitual low calcium communities can thrive.

Here are the snags of the useful minerals:

CALCIUM
Calcium overdose has been observed both in infants and adults. The cause is a combination of excess absorption caused by the infants being given too much vitamin D, or the adults taking too much; and the individuals being extra-sensitive to vitamin D. Although the ill-effects are serious – with permanent damage or death in infants – the condition is very rare. For the vast majority of people, the body will simply dispense with any calcium beyond what it needs for body repairs.

CHROMIUM
Chromium is never eaten to excess in foods. Chromium can be an industrial waste pollutant, which accumulates in the lungs in an insoluble form.

COBALT

Cobalt overdose may cause enlargement of the thyroid gland, an effect usually due to a deficiency of iodine. This would not usually happen unless extra amounts of the element were taken deliberately – something there is no reason to do. Supplements are not sold, and we should eat foods which supply plenty of vitamin B12 (and cobalt automatically comes with it).

COPPER

Copper overdose is potentially one of the most common in our society, thanks to several 'new' factors in our lives.

Oestrogen elevates the body level of copper in a copper containing protein – and oestrogen in the form of oral contraceptives or hormone replacement at menopause is taken by about three million women in the U.K. alone.

Copper water piping can result in far higher than normal levels of the mineral in our drinking water, especially in areas where the water supply is naturally acidic. Don't drink water from the hot water taps, or use it in the kettle or for cooking.

Zinc and copper are antagonistic, and a high intake of copper may depress body zinc levels.

The ill-effects of excess copper in such amounts are not clearly defined, but it has been stated by Carl Pfeiffer that blood copper levels are high in those who have died from early heart attacks, in patients with high blood pressure, and in smokers. The genetic Wilson's disease, where the body is unable to dispense with unwanted copper and stores it in the brain and liver producing mental illness, cirrhosis of the liver or Parkinsonism are fortunately rare, and can now be arrested by giving the sufferer substances which combine with the stored copper, and enable the body to excrete it. People with Wilson's disease in the family need to alert their doctor even if they have no symptoms.

FLUORIDE

Fluoride is very easily toxic in excess, and such excess is unusual in occurring in the water of some areas naturally. Communities where the fluoride content of the water is over four or five parts per million tend to have mottled teeth, with bands of brown and white.

More severe poisoning has been seen in some places in Argentina, China and India, where the water contains over ten parts per million of fluoride. This level (which could also occur among workers handling fluoride-carrying minerals used to smelt aluminium) causes the skeleton to become rigid and inflexible, as the bones become denser. The amount of fluoride added to water in some areas to try to reduce tooth decay is one part per million. However, even this amount, Dr Dean Burk in America alleges, has raised cancer deaths substantially in a number of areas of the U.S.A. with fluoridated water, which he has compared with non-fluoridated water supply areas.

His views are very controversial, but the move to fluoridate water has halted in several countries as a result of general doubt about the safety of the measure. Since the cause of tooth decay is not lack of fluoride, but eating sugary foods, no one need worry that they should take fluoride tablets, even though these are at a low dosage.

If you live in a fluoridated water area, and do not want to take extra fluoride, it has recently become possible to buy a filter which will remove it. Previously, only a distiller would do this job, and distillation leaves water without any beneficial minerals and unpleasant to drink. The new filter was developed by Doulton Products* (a sister company of Royal Doulton) for the Dutch government who wanted to give householders the opportunity of opting out of fluoridation before the element was added to the national water supply. Then the Dutch decided against fluoridating their water at all – but

* Doulton Industrial Products Ltd., Stone, Staffs. ST15 0PU.

the filter is now available. It is not attached to a household tap, and is used only for water which will be drunk or used in cooking. You pour water in at the top, it filters through special charcoal into a container at the bottom with a little tap, storing two gallons at a time. Every few months, depending on the amount of water used, the charcoal is replaced with more from a refill pack.

IODINE

Iodine is not toxic in the amounts available in food, but can be in supplement form and cannot be bought in supplement form over the counter.

IRON

Iron excess from food does not occur, as most people obtain barely enough, and excess is excreted.

HAZARDS TO HEALTH

The second group of minerals is far more sinister. It consists of those that you don't need or want in your body at all. Three such minerals are cadmium, lead and mercury. They are all 'heavy metals' which reach us as a consequence of industrialization, and they are real hazards to health.

CADMIUM

Sweden and Japan have both provided cases of serious cadmium poisoning. Prolonged contact with the metal via water, food or air causes a painful and potentially fatal disease which the Japanese call *itai itai* disease.

It happened in Sweden in the 1930's and 40's at a factory where the production of cadmium and nickel electrodes left cadmium fumes and dust in the air. It happened in Japan where mines released waste material heavy with cadmium into a river. The people who lived downstream drank water and ate rice grown with the water that was polluted. In both cases the effects were severe: kidney damage being the most outstanding, followed by painful softening of the bones.

We all encounter cadmium every day. We meet it

in the air: it is estimated that about 0.02 micrograms are inhaled daily by an adult. This is a very small amount compared to other sources, but smokers take in many many times more and they have been found to have far higher levels of the mineral in their livers and kidneys.

More cadmium comes from food. Nearly all foods contain a little, but if the soil or water of an area has been polluted every vegetable grown there and every animal reared there will be affected. As liver and kidney are the body's storage zones, they will be the main places where the cadmium will accumulate. Also, oysters are especially vulnerable to the absorption of the mineral from polluted waters. So, the main items to avoid in a cadmium-heavy region are kidneys, liver and oysters.

Unfortunately, no one has yet found an agent which enables the body to rid itself of excess cadmium faster than normal such as has been found for copper and lead excess. However, it is clear that deficiencies of other elements can increase the accumulation and harmfulness of cadmium. Ones which have been identified as cadmium-antagonists are calcium, copper, iron, protein, vitamin D and zinc. Natural, unprocessed foods which are good sources of such elements are therefore our best protection since the amount of cadmium in our environment is usually outside our control – unless we smoke.

LEAD

The dangers of lead are among the few environmental hazards that almost everyone is aware of. Recently attention has been focussed on lead as a cause of disturbed behaviour among children living near motorway junctions. However, the risks have neither been thoroughly researched nor widely publicized by the authorities; perhaps because the results would force action on a very difficult political issue: petrol. This, or rather exhaust fumes, is the main source of lead pollution. Although it contains less than can be found in food, we absorb more effectively through our lungs than intestinal walls.

The second contributor is old lead water piping which can still be in use in houses over sixty years old. And third on the list comes the lead solder used on food cans. So, all of us are exposed to lead pollution regularly, and even small amounts of this metal can have bad effects. However, these tend to be so generalized as to be almost never traced back to lead pollution as the cause. The most common symptoms are headaches, dizziness, irritability, insomnia, muscle weakness or spasms and, when exposure is heightened, anaemia, for one of the most serious effects of lead is to hinder the formation of new blood cells.

There is little we can do to influence directly the amount of lead in our environment short of joining one of the pressure groups, but there are some things we can do to limit our exposure. Firstly, stop smoking. Secondly, check water pipes and if they are lead, either have them changed or use a water filter, or buy spring water in bottles for drinking. A good tip is to run the tap a while before drawing drinking water, especially first thing in the morning. What you eat matters too, and fortunately good nutrition protects against lead absorption to some extent.

MERCURY

Mercury poisoning has happened often enough to provide us with plenty of evidence of its effects. Compounds of mercury such as methyl mercury reach us via dressings used as fungicides on grain; via fish which collect mercury from contaminated waters. Japan is again an example, and the poisoning in their Minamata region resulted in the disease caused being named after it.

Apart from evading mercury contamination which comes from a job involving the metal, there is little the individual can do to avoid pollution. But, again, the better the general health and level of nutrition, the less likely ill-effects are.

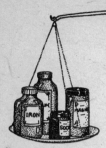
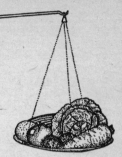

CHAPTER TWELVE

WHERE DO YOU STAND?

How can you find out whether your supply of
minerals is adequate, or which minerals your body
contains too much or too little of? Current
technology provides no satisfactory answer to this
question. No one worries about mineral status unless
symptoms of ill-health become obvious, and only
recently have the characteristic mineral
abnormalities attached to such conditions as women
taking oral contraceptives, or schizophrenics been
studied.

Poisoning from lead or other heavy metals will be
spotted by your doctor once it is clearly making you
ill; and iron-deficiency anaemia, iodine deficiency
or calcium shortages are all regularly detected – but
only when their progress is far enough advanced to
be uncomfortable.

UNDETECTED DEFICIENCIES
Small deficiencies can easily go undetected for years.
There are two, interlinked, reasons for this less-than-
reassuring position. The first is that looking to
minerals for an explanation of illness is a very new
idea. It is not a very acceptable idea yet, given the

common medical view that most people are well nourished, and certainly will not be short of a substance that is needed by the body in amounts you could fit on a pinhead.

Yet the same orthodox world recognizes deficiencies of iodine and vitamin B12 – involving just as tiny amounts – because they produce distinctive ill-effects.

So it is just a question of time before more observation is made of the effects of small and large deficiencies of other trace elements, which may not show so obviously. At present, zinc is receiving this kind of detailed attention in several countries. Let us hope it turns out that few symptoms of ill-health in our society are due to mineral deficiency, but that some answers to current health problems are found.

The second, linked, reason for lack of attention to minerals is that until the last fifteen or twenty years, techniques for measuring minerals, particularly trace elements, either did not exist or were crude.

ASSESSING MINERAL STATUS

There is still debate about the best way to obtain an accurate picture of the body's mineral status. Analyses of blood, urine and hair are the methods used, with hair gaining appreciation as a method only recently. The attraction of hair analysis is that it gives a more static picture of the body's mineral stores. Blood and urine samples can rise and fall within short periods of time.

If you suspect that you are suffering from a mineral imbalance, the first thing to do is to tell your doctor or other practitioner what symptoms you are suffering from, or why you think mineral imbalance is present. Do not be embarrassed by the assumption that your doctor will dismiss your anxieties as neuroses. He may, but that is his problem rather than yours. He is still committed to trying to find out what he can about your situation. Many doctors will not dismiss your anxieties lightly. In any case, going to your doctor is the only way to get access to diagnostic tests without paying extra for them.

SPECTROPHOTOMETRY

There is another avenue to finding out your mineral status, and one that is open to you even if you have no signs of ill-health and are just curious to know where you stand. This is to send a sample of your head hair to a laboratory which specializes in hair analysis for minerals. A leading laboratory carrying out this type of work is Albion Laboratories, in Utah, U.S.A. They analyse thousands of hair samples each year, sent in by doctors or members of the public.

The hair must come from within one inch of the scalp to give a true reflection of mineral status. Most people cut it from the nape of the neck. Three full tablespoonsful are needed. The hair should not have been treated with dyes or conditioners for a full month before cutting, and Albion only accept hair from the head. This is because they have worked out how this represents overall mineral status. Hair from the arms, legs, chest, etc., could have a different relationship.

Albion carry out analyses for most minerals, the cost rising with the number of tests made. An analyses for eight main minerals, plus lead, costs in the region of £17. For this, you receive a computer printout sheet showing on a chart how your levels of each mineral compare with normal ranges of that mineral in men and women. The chart also indicates how the minerals which affect one another stand, in terms of 'too low relative to calcium', for instance. The minerals which are strikingly high or low are also picked out. All this helps the recipient judge his position, and what he might do about it.

The method Albion use is called *spectrophotometry* and is the only accepted method at present. However, you may well see advertisements in the press for another kind of mineral analysis. The offer is that you send a lock of hair to a given address with a fee, and receive back a mineral (and also perhaps a vitamin) analysis. The people offering such services believe that individuals with special sympathetic powers can analyse your mineral status (and lots more about you) just from a piece of hair. They may use a pendulum.

You may believe that this is a worthwhile service. That is up to you. This author does not.

If your doctor detects some mineral deficiency (iron is the commonest), he will provide prescriptions for treatment or not, according to his judgement.

TAKING MINERAL SUPPLEMENTS

If you obtain a hair analysis independently, you will have guidelines to follow in taking supplements. There is little to choose between most of the mineral supplements on the market, in today's state of limited knowledge about ideal dosages and formulations. The exception is chelated minerals, which have been shown to be more efficiently absorbed. This is a help if the problem is poor absorption, not poor supply.

Whatever minerals you take, do not expect them to work like magic 'wonder drugs'. As with most natural treatments, patience is needed, and you should take a bottleful (at the rate recommended on the label) before expecting to notice any difference. Effects can be more rapid, but persevere if they are not.

Remember too that supplements are no replacement for eating the right food. Upgrade your eating habits to bring more mineral-rich foods into your daily life – and you will be investing in a more soundly mineralized future.

SOURCES OF MINERALS YOU COULD RUN SHORT OF

Calcium Dairy products, fresh green leafy vegetables, oily fish.

Chromium Beef, beer, molasses, brewer's yeast, grape juice, offal, wholegrains.

Cobalt Almost exclusive to animal foods, i.e. meat, fish, dairy foods, eggs.

Iodine Sea fish, shellfish, seaweed, fish liver oils, iodized salt.

Iron Black pudding, offal meats, game, shellfish, soya

beans, dried apricots, sardines, molasses, beef, lamb, dark green vegetables.

Magnesium Seafood, wheat germ, nuts, beans, wholegrain cereals, leafy green vegetables

Molybdenum Not known – so a general, varied and unprocessed diet is suggested.

Potassium Dried fruit, especially prunes, soya flour, fruit juices, expecially citrus, potatoes, molasses, nuts, fruit, cider vinegar.

Selenium Seafood, meat, seaweed.

Silicon Unrefined cereals, beer.

Sulphur Protein foods, both animal and vegetable.

Vanadium Unrefined cereals, nuts, root vegetables.

Zinc Seafood, meat, whole grains, nuts, pulses.

SUMMARY

Some foods are clearly top of the league as providers of minerals. Seafoods – both fish and seaweed products such as kelp, caragean, agar agar, laver and dulse – are rich sources of a variety of elements. Vegetarians can obtain ample if less concentrated supplies from vegetables, especially the leafy dark green varieties, and from fresh fruit. Nuts and pulses are sources of many useful minerals. Fats, sugar and refined cereals are poor providers of minerals.

Thus the health-conscious person will concentrate on these unprocessed foods, and should then fulfil all normal requirements for minerals. Apart from their individual value, eating minerals in natural balance is more likely to produce a happy combination than does concentrating on supplements or on one or two particular foods.